Child Public Health

Mitch Blair

Reader in Paediatrics and Child Public Health, Imperial College London and Northwick Park Hospital, Harrow

Sarah Stewart–Brown

Professor of Public Health, Warwick Medical School, Warwick University

Tony Waterston

Consultant Paediatrician, Newcastle General Hospital, Newcastle-upon-Tyne

Rachel Crowther

Specialist Registrar in Public Health, Department of Public Health and Primary Care, University of Oxford

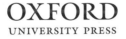

OXFORD
UNIVERSITY PRESS

OXFORD
UNIVERSITY PRESS

Great Clarendon Street, Oxford OX2 6DP

Oxford University Press is a department of the University of Oxford.
It furthers the University's objective of excellence in research, scholarship,
and education by publishing worldwide in

Oxford New York

Auckland Cape Town Dar es Salaam Hong Kong Karachi
Kuala Lumpur Madrid Melbourne Mexico City Nairobi
New Delhi Shanghai Taipei Toronto

With offices in

Argentina Austria Brazil Chile Czech Republic France Greece
Guatemala Hungary Italy Japan South Korea Poland Portugal
Singapore Switzerland Thailand Turkey Ukraine Vietnam

Published in the United States
by Oxford University Press Inc., New York

A catalogue record for this title is available from the British Library

ISBN 978 0 19 263192 3 (Pbk)

10 9 8 7 6 5

Typeset by Newgen Imaging Systems (P) Ltd., Chennai, India
Printed in Great Britain
on acid-free paper by
Biddles Ltd., King's Lynn, Norfolk

Child Public Health

To our parents and our children:
"*From whence we came, we go.*"

And in affectionate and grateful memory of Professor David Baum, the first President of the Royal College of Paediatrics and Child Health.

Foreword

David Hall

When clinicians begin their training in hospital paediatrics they are generally fascinated by the diagnostic and technical challenges of caring for sick children – and so they should be. But as experience grows, one begins to appreciate that many of the children who are admitted or who attend clinics have preventable disorders. The over-representation of children from run-down communities, and the extent of the psychological distress and social disruption that are the lot of many children, only gradually intrude on one's awareness.

If that is the experience of professionals training in the privileged Western world, how much more so is it true in poor countries where the vast majority of the illnesses seen in a children's ward are entirely preventable. The personal journey that begins with the care of an individual sick child takes one first into the territory of preventive measures like immunisation and clean water and ultimately to more fundamental issues of poverty, exploitation and inequality.

Can that journey be accelerated – and would this be a good idea? Of course, the majority of those who embark on paediatric training will spend most of their careers in clinical practice. But even the most specialised clinician should be asking themselves – why is this child here? Was this condition (and this admission) preventable? Does this child represent the tip of an iceberg of pathology in the community? What are the social circumstances from which he comes and to which he will return? How might they be relevant to his care?

For some professionals, public health questions soon become the main focus of their career. They will want to know about the strengths and weaknesses, the health and the illness profile, and the resources, that characterise the community for which they are responsible. And of course, they will want to know how they can make a difference.

Whatever one's interests, children's public health is not an easy subject to study. While some of the underpinning sciences, such as epidemiology and statistics, are well described in many texts, an overview of the political and cultural context in which public health is practised is more difficult to find. The authors of this book have set out to give us just such an overview and they have succeeded admirably. Those with community – wide responsibilities will be delighted with the many practical examples and analyses. But there is no longer any excuse for any child health professional, however specialised, to plead ignorance of the subject.

Foreword

Sian Griffiths

This book emphasizes the importance of child public health as a rapidly emerging field and puts the health of children centre stage as society's greatest asset. It maps out what needs to be done to promote and protect the health of children not only in the UK, but internationally.

Health is not the absence of disease but a more complex interaction between social, physical, environmental, and psychological factors which contribute to wellness and well-being. Healthy children are not merely the product of a good healthcare system. Although children and young people themselves are of central importance, they need to be seen within the context of their families, communities, environments, and wider social and political settings. As the authors stress, it is not possible to improve the health of children without addressing social policy, family relationships, environmental concerns, and community structures. These are all central concerns of those interested in child public health—a re-emerging subspecialty of public health and paediatrics which combines concern for promoting health, preventing disease, and ensuring quality services for children and young people. Central to the approach of child public health is the concern not only for the individual child but also for populations of children and young people, in both developed countries and across the developing world.

One of the key concerns of any caring society must be to address social inequalities which manifest themselves through higher rates of illness and death amongst children coming from more deprived backgrounds. Throughout this book, society's responsibility to ensure a good start in life for children is stressed, to enable them to be as free as possible from disease, disability, and distress with their wishes and needs understood and respected. Child public health stresses the need not only for a better understanding of upstream intervention within the health service but for partnership and collaboration with teachers, social workers, youth workers, and others in the community whose work and policies can promote young people's health.

Tracing the history of community child health reminds us that whilst major threats to child health in developed countries such as the UK reflect the diseases of affluence, many parts of the world still face the ravages of infectious disease and poverty not dissimilar to those seen through the eyes of commentators such as Dickens a century ago. 85% of the world's children live in developing countries and the importance of the international context of child health is described in some detail, emphasizing the global nature of issues of higher rates of infectious disease and illness related to poor nutrition, at the same time as facing the epidemics of the developed world, obesity, diabetes, and heart disease.

The obesity epidemic in developed countries serves as a reminder of the need for effective evidence based interventions. Any professional group needs to be clear about the skills and competencies expected from its practitioners and specialists. Child public health is no exception and this book spells out the underlying science behind the specialty including basic epidemiological concepts and discussion about evidence and its use. It also provides practical examples through scenarios which reflect common problems. The book acts as a wake-up call to both paediatrics and public health, reminding us of our responsibilities to children within communities— for promoting their health as well as delivering their health care. These responsibilities need to be taken seriously.

Contents

Introduction

Why child public health?

Who is this book for?

For well over a century policy makers and medical professionals alike have understood the importance of child health for society. Healthy children grow up into strong, healthy, fulfilled, and productive adults, able themselves to nurture the next generation and carry society forwards—but we have also come to realise that ensuring that our children are healthy and happy is an important end in itself. The right of children to enjoy childhood to the fullest extent possible is enshrined in the United Nations Convention on the Rights of the Child as well as in the legal framework of many countries. Children make up around 20% of the UK population, and as much as 50% in some other countries. They are a vulnerable group, politically disempowered as non-voters with no formal civic representation. They need others to advocate for them and to ensure their rights—including the right to health—are protected.

Child public health involves promoting the health and well-being of young people in the widest sense. It is an endeavour which requires the commitment and co-operation of a wide range of individuals and organizations: health, social care, and education professionals; local and national government, including departments of transport, housing, and leisure; the voluntary sector, at local, national, and international levels; the police force, legal, and criminal justice systems; and of course children and young people themselves, and their parents, families, friends, and carers. This book is for all of them. It aims to support all health care professionals interested in the health of children and young people, especially those working or training in the fields of public health, primary care, and paediatrics. It also provides an introduction to the principles and practice of child public health for everyone with an interest in the subject—from doctors to social workers and teachers, and from parents and voluntary workers to probation officers.

For those working in child health in both community and hospital settings, this book aims to explore the preventive aspects of clinical practice, demonstrating the importance of public health principles both in everyday practice and in the planning of future services. For the public health professional with a wide portfolio to address, it seeks to highlight some of the public health issues specific to children which are common and amenable to the approaches described in later chapters. Primary health care teams are being given an increasingly important role in the modern NHS with regard to health needs assessment and the commissioning of services for their population. This text will appeal to primary care professionals with an interest in children's health and will help them with these responsibilities. Because mental health is such a key issue for child health today the book will also be of value to professionals working in child and adolescent mental health services who have an interest in prevention.

Some of the material will be familiar to some readers, but the aim is to bridge a number of divides—between branches of the medical profession, between different professions and disciplines, between the statutory and voluntary sectors, and between the professional and lay perspective. We hope that there will be something here to interest and inform every reader.

Whilst the book has been written by people working in the UK and uses mainly UK examples of public health practice, the global perspective is well recognized, and the principles and approaches espoused are relevant to those practising or intending to practice child public health throughout the developed world.

What is child public health?

The concept of health, and the definition of public health, are complex issues which are dealt with in some detail in Chapter 4. It will become clear that child public health is neither a single nor a simple entity, and that it involves a range of ideals, activities, and academic disciplines. It covers the study of patterns of health and illness in children and young people, the various factors which affect their health, and the ways in which we—as individuals, organizations, professions, and societies—can modify these factors in order to improve the health and well-being of all young people. Kohler's definition provides a useful starting point, describing child public health as:

> ...the organised efforts of society to develop healthy public health policies to promote child and young people's health, to prevent disease in children and young people and to foster equity for children and young people, within a framework of sustainable development.

We have chosen not to define precisely what we mean by a child, nor to divide up this book into sections according to the various age groups which make up childhood and adolescence. This is partly because we perceive the process of growing up as a continuous one, so that drawing a sharp line between a child and an adult is unhelpful. Although the patterns of ill health and of factors influencing health shift as a child gets older, many of the important determinants of child health, and resulting health problems, affect children and young people at several different stages of development. This book is structured on a more thematic basis, recognizing the need to act across a range of ages, sectors, and professional boundaries. It takes an inclusive approach which covers children from conception through to the teenage years and the transition to adulthood.

Although children and young people themselves are of central importance, it is essential to see them in context—within their families, communities, environments, and wider social and political setting. All these constitute layers of influence on the individual child and the child population, and spheres of activity for child public health practice. We cannot hope to improve the lot of children and young people, now or in the future, without addressing social policy, family relationships, environmental concerns, and community structures.

Why is child public health important?

Child public health is emerging—or perhaps re-emerging—as a subspecialty of both public health and paediatrics, and as a broadly based interdisciplinary movement. We have already hinted at some of the reasons why this is a welcome and an important development and why, therefore, we feel the need to devote a whole book to public health with a child focus.

Defining a common interest

As a secondary interest of many professionals but the particular focus of few, child public health has tended until recently to fall between several different stools. Most current public health literature and action addresses the proportionately (and literally!) larger adult population. Very few public health professionals have a predominantly child health focus, perhaps with the exception of health visitors and school nurses.

Many of those working in paediatrics and general practice tend to focus on personal health services and interventions at the level of the individual, and are not used to considering problems or solutions at community or population level. Most have, however, noticed considerable changes in their case loads and the problems presenting to them over the last few decades, changes which reflect social, economic, and political factors as well as medical ones, and which need to be tackled both at population level and through individual consultations.

The public health and clinical approaches are often considered to be qualitatively different ways of responding to health and disease, with the former focussing on the population and the latter on the individual—or the one 'upstream', concerned with the causes and determinants of ill health, and the other 'downstream', dealing with the consequences. In practice, many child health workers combine the individual and population perspectives in their day-to-day work and share a similar aim—that of optimizing the health and well-being of all children and young people. Defining common ground, and understanding what those with different backgrounds can contribute to the common cause, is an important objective of child public health.

But the need for common understanding and co-operation goes much wider than the health sector. Many teachers, social workers, educational psychologists, and others working with children in a variety of disciplines are becoming increasingly aware that health and behaviour problems impinge on and are affected by factors within their own spheres of operation, but may feel they lack the means—or indeed the time—to engage with others in order to address them.

There is a need to draw together all these perspectives into a coherent movement which tackles the health and health-related problems of children. Those working with children across different disciplines need to act together on the broader determinants of child health. This means acquiring new knowledge and skills and working in new ways, and this book aims to provide some of the necessary information and tools.

Understanding and responding to changes in child health

There has been a major shift in the patterns of morbidity and mortality (ill health and death) over the past century in developed countries, and it is important to understand the reasons for these changes and to respond to them.

As the burden of perinatal mortality, infectious disease, and malnutrition has declined, there has been an increase in multifactorial disorders and conditions which require a more complex therapeutic approach. These include mental, emotional, and behavioural problems, physical and neurodevelopmental disabilities, teenage pregnancy, and child abuse. These are often referred to as the 'new' morbidities and they require an eclectic approach and set of skills in order to tackle them. Another of the key objectives of child public health is to explore and elucidate changes in health and disease in children, to provide those concerned with the tools needed to assess the health problems and needs of their child population, and to provide guidance on appropriate ways of meeting them.

Child health as an end in itself and as a major determinant of adult health

Children in their own right deserve the best possible health and protection from harmful influences. The United Nations Convention on the Rights of the Child enshrines many important principles of child public health, including the right of children to health, safety, identity—and to be heard and listened to. As a society, we have a responsibility to ensure that children have as good a start in life as we can give them, and can enjoy their early years as free as they can be from disease, disability, and distress, with their wishes and needs understood and respected.

In particular, we have a responsibility towards less advantaged children in this and other countries—children whose rights are more likely to be infringed and whose health, development, and self-expression is more likely to be compromised. Inequalities in health are, as we shall see, particularly marked in children: those from the lowest social class have twice the chance of dying before their first birthday as those from the highest social class, and almost all illnesses and causes of death are more common in poorer and socially excluded children. The collective endeavour which is child public health has a role to play in safeguarding children's rights, tackling health inequalities in children, and ensuring that children's health is kept at the forefront in social policy, health care planning, and our national (and international) conscience.

Recent research has illuminated the contribution which physical and emotional factors in infancy and childhood make to adult health and disease. This has added additional impetus to research on child health and to the development of disease prevention and health promotion initiatives among children as future adults.

Pioneers in child public health

A number of pioneering individuals from different professional backgrounds have brought a public health perspective to bear on child health problems over the last couple of centuries, making significant contributions to the health and well-being of children and setting examples of the wide sphere of influence of child public health interventions. Some of their work is described below.

One of the earliest pioneers of child public health, Edward Jenner (1749–1823), a Gloucestershire country physician, made the important observation that milkmaids who had contracted cowpox seemed to be immune from catching smallpox. Jenner inoculated a small boy, James Phepps, with cowpox material by scratching it onto his arm, and then proceeded to test his hypothesis by inoculating him with smallpox. The discovery that James was indeed protected from smallpox heralded the era of vaccination and the later development of what remains one of the most successful preventive measures available to the medical profession.

James Spence (1892–1954) was the first Professor of Child Health (as opposed to clinical paediatrics) in England and set up the first babies' hospital where mothers could 'room in' (stay in the hospital with their children). His survey of the causes of infant mortality in the North East, undertaken with the co-operation of the city councils, was one of the first population-based (as opposed to hospital-based) investigations carried out by a paediatrician. He took a similar 'community approach' with

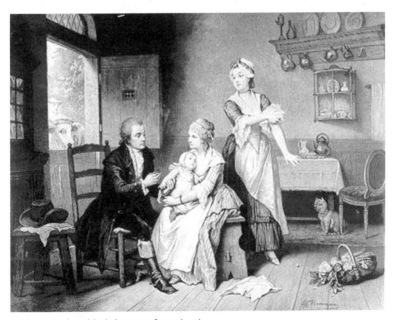

Edward Jenner heralded the era of vaccination

the establishment of the 'Thousand Families' project, which followed up all babies born in May and June of 1947. This was one of the first studies to show clearly the association between poverty and ill health. It was also one of the first studies to show that the ill effects of poverty could be traced from one generation to another in intergenerational cycles of disadvantage.

Donald Court succeeded James Spence on his death, and was influential for his recognition of the importance of community paediatric services, and for his calls to strengthen the study of social determinants of health and disease in the child and family. Court ensured that these factors were included in the education of health professionals. He chaired the UK Commission of Enquiry into the Child Health Services, 'Fit for the Future', which reported in 1976 and recommended the establishment of multidisciplinary teams, integrated community and hospital paediatric services, and primary paediatric care delivered by GPs. Court always maintained that preventive medicine should be given the same status as curative medicine:

> Without continuing enquiry, there is no progression. My plea is that we should apply the same critical energy to the study of social as we do to cellular behaviour.

In the USA, Abraham Jacobi (1830–1919) was a radical socialist paediatrician, the first Professor in the Diseases of Children in the US, and President of the American Medical Association. He made careful studies of the causes of infant mortality and was a great advocate for the promotion of breast-feeding, especially amongst the poor of New York. He called for the development of high-quality maternity services and midwifery schools and was amongst the first to speak out against artificial milk manufacturers, mocking the advertising of the time. In 1912, Nestlé produced a poster of a woman with immense wings, perhaps representing an angel, which Jacobi described as if 'flying off with two babies to unknown parts', alluding to the increased infant death rates from artificial feeding. He recognized the need for doctors to:

> ... enlighten and direct public opinion in regard to the broad problems of hygiene, and of representing to the world the practical accomplishments of scientific medicine.

During the 1870s, Jacobi set up summer corps of doctors to work in the tenements of New York—a case of positive discrimination in health service provision towards those most in need. In later decades, he was heavily involved in the formation of the Society for the Prevention of Cruelty to Children and other welfare organizations.

Charles Dickens is another influential figure in promoting child public health in the nineteenth century. In his writings he gave a vivid picture of the plight of children living in poor social circumstances. His attention to detail often caused shock and disbelief in his public readings of his works. Through his novels and serials, in particular *Oliver Twist* and *David Copperfield*, he was able to describe the effects of the Industrial Revolution and the immense social changes of the nineteenth century. His work as an advocate for children was recognized in his invitation to speak at the opening of the Hospital for Sick Children in Great Ormond Street, London.

Another non-medical pioneer in child public health was Edwin Chadwick (1800–1890), Secretary to the Poor Law Commissioners. Together with Anthony Cooper,

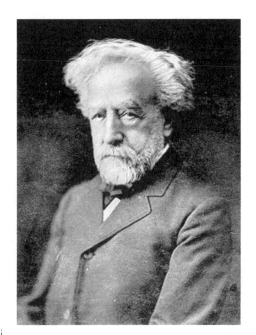

Abraham Jacobi

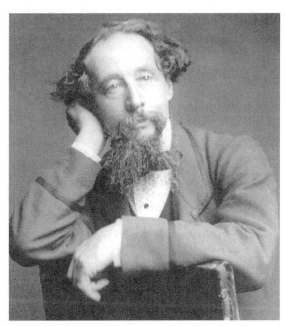

Charles Dickens (from Ackroyd, P. *Dickens: Public Life and Private Passion*. BBC Books)

the Seventh Earl of Shaftesbury, he was instrumental in protecting the well-being of children by limiting the age at which they could be legally employed in the factories and mills of the time. The Factory Act of 1833 excluded children under the age of nine from working in factories, limited work by children under fourteen to 48 hours per week, and made provision for this same group to attend school for at least two hours a day. Opponents to the Act were deeply concerned that the industrial welfare of the country would be severely threatened by the loss of two hours per day of up to 30,000 girl workers, fearing that 'our manufacturing supremacy would depart from us'.

Chadwick also authored a major review of the sanitary condition of the labouring classes in England and Wales which was published in 1842. Amongst the recommendations he made were the development of water and sanitation supplies to the major towns—a public health measure to help prevent the cholera epidemics which were then sweeping the world with massive infant and child mortality in their wake. It is easy to forget that at this time, four out of five houses in Birmingham and eleven out of twelve in Newcastle had no water supply. Chadwick was said to be a harsh, domineering man, but he had the qualities of persistence and tenacity often required to make fundamental changes in social policy.

John Snow (1813–58) is also remembered for his historic contribution to tackling cholera. During the London cholera epidemic of 1854, in which over five hundred people died in ten days within a radius of 250 yards of Broad Street, Snow's meticulous geographical plotting of the cases, and exploration of their water supply, led to the conclusion that the Broad Street water pump was the source of the disease and to the removal of the pump handle to prevent further cases. Snow's work, though not directly concerned with child health, had an important indirect impact on childhood diseases. The famous episode of the Broad Street pump contributed significantly to the evidence for infectious agents as specific causes of disease, thus opening the door to the treatment and prevention of the infectious diseases which constituted a major cause of mortality and morbidity in children at the time.

The structure of this book

The rest of this book is divided into seven chapters. The first two set the scene, both in the UK and worldwide. They should be of interest to all readers, although some of the material will be familiar to those working in paediatrics and public health. The first chapter describes the major determinants of health and the current patterns of ill health in children in the UK, reflecting on the main changes which have occurred in recent decades, and setting out the key challenges for child public health today. The second chapter goes on to highlight the very different child health problems facing developing countries, many of them related to poverty, and outlines the significant connection and interdependence which exists between the developed and developing worlds. This chapter aims to provide a global perspective for child health in the UK and suggests that international child health should be a matter of concern for us all.

Chapter 1

Child health in the UK

This chapter addresses the health and well-being of children in the UK today. It looks at the impact of the far-reaching changes of the last 50 years—in the family and socioeconomic environment, food and nutrition, transport, lifestyle, and communications technology—and identifies the major child health problems at the start of the twenty-first century.

Children in the UK

The population of children and young people (aged 0–19 years) in Great Britain at the end of the twentieth century was just over 14.5 million. Britain is a relatively small and a very prosperous country, and modern media and information technology have done much to universalize the experience of young people. Despite these facts, British children are not a homogeneous group. Their life experiences, and the problems they face, vary substantially. Socio-economic and geographical differences account for much of the difference, and social factors such as intolerance and stigma, family relationships, and employment practices are also highly significant.

Almost 1.5 million children and young people in the UK are from an ethnic minority group.

Children living in rural communities—some of them remote—have very different lives from those growing up in inner cities. Children's domestic lives also vary, and the patterns of family composition are changing. The number of dependent children living in one-parent families in Great Britain increased from 1 million to 2.8

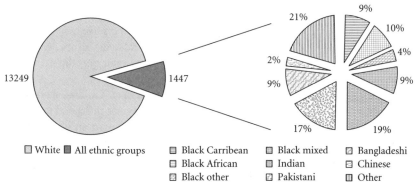

Fig. 1.1 Ethnic composition of children aged 0–14 in England and Wales 1998/9. (Source: ONS.)

million between 1961 and 1996. Nearly a quarter of households with dependent children now have only one parent. Most children still live in households where children are hit by adults. At the same time, the 'Watch with Mother' culture of the 1960s has given way to one in which many preschool children spend significant amounts of time in day care facilities.

The changing pattern of children's health

A time traveller from a previous century would probably conclude that most children in the UK today are extremely healthy and that most of their needs are met. Although this is not the whole story, it is certainly the case that on many counts child health has improved dramatically in the last century (see Chapter 3). Child mortality and morbidity have fallen dramatically, children are growing taller, they are participating more in society, disease and disability are better treated, and there are better and more focussed services for preschool children. Improvements have been achieved in the treatment of childhood cancer, in mortality and morbidity from accidents, and of course in the prevention and treatment of infectious diseases. There is no doubt that we have much to be proud of and that UK children are healthier than at almost any time in the past. This is due largely to improved nutrition, housing, smaller families, water and sewage treatment, and also to the beneficial effects of immunization.

Yet the perceptive time traveller would also notice a new set of child health problems, some of which may not be manifest until later in life. The UK has one of the highest levels of relative child poverty in Europe, and this has wide-ranging consequences for health. Emotional and behavioural problems are increasingly pervasive. Teachers in inner-city schools report difficulties in controlling children's behaviour even in the reception class, and many older children are beyond the control of their parents. Truancy rates are increasing, and newspapers carry stories about crimes committed by children as young as 10 or 11. Obesity in childhood is rising sharply; more young people are committing suicide; smoking and binge drinking are at epidemic proportions in teenagers. Children watch more and more television, and the use of mobile phones is increasing dramatically. Both these phenomena significantly affect their patterns of social interaction and have health consequences. We have the highest teenage pregnancy and sexually transmitted infection rates in Europe, and child pedestrians in the UK are at significantly greater risk of injury on the roads than those in the rest of Northern Europe.

Recently, inequalities in child health have been increasing. Children from lower social classes have a much greater chance of dying in infancy or childhood than those from higher social classes. Babies whose mothers were born in Pakistan, the Caribbean, and Africa (except East Africa) have higher mortality throughout infancy. In 1989–91, the perinatal mortality rate for infants of mothers born in Pakistan was almost double the rate of the UK-born mothers. However, infants of Asian- and African-born mothers have lower rates of sudden infant death syndrome than those of UK-born mothers.

Certain groups of children—including children of asylum seekers, those with disabilities, and the socially excluded—fail to benefit from the opportunities available to others in society. Up to 20% of UK children are considered to be vulnerable or in need (see box).

Vulnerable children—children who would benefit from extra help from public agencies to optimize their life chances and for the risk of social exclusion to be averted. They include:

- Children in public care
- Children with disabilities
- Pupils with behaviour and attendance problems
- Children in need of protection
- Children in need of family support
- Young offenders
- Young carers
- Children and adolescents with mental health problems
- Young drug misusers
- Teenage parents
- Children of asylum seekers

Children in need—a subset of vulnerable children including children in need of protection, family support, or in public care.

These children often have a very different experience of life—and of health—from their peers.

The emergence of these new child health problems reflects the change in UK society as a whole over the past 50 years. Although many of these problems present to health professionals, including GPs, paediatricians, health visitors, school nurses, and child psychiatrists, these are problems which cannot be solved by health services alone. As this chapter will illustrate, their causes lie in a wide range of social, economic, and environmental factors, and in order to tackle them action is needed across just as broad a spectrum. Professionals in other voluntary and statutory agencies (including education, social services, probation, and the police) encounter the same problems, and have a shared interest in addressing them. The public health approach—assessing and grappling with the determinants of health through joint working with a wide range of agencies and the involvement of communities—is essential if we are to make any headway. Many of these problems are examined in more detail throughout the course of this book, and the final chapter will explore the application of the public health perspective to their solution.

Key messages

- Changing pattern of children's health
- Better nutrition and fewer infectious diseases
- Relative poverty is increasing
- More mental health problems, teenage pregnancy, obesity, drug taking, and smoking
- Accidents still a major cause of death
- A public health approach to these problems is essential

Measuring health and disease

Despite the importance of viewing health as a positive concept rather than as merely the absence of disease (see Chapter 4), it is diseases and health problems which are generally measured when statistics are collected. Much of the information in this section thus relates not to health but to the absence of health.

Mortality in infancy and childhood has fallen significantly over the last century. Improvements in the prevention and treatment of infectious diseases have been highly significant in this fall in childhood mortality, but other factors have played

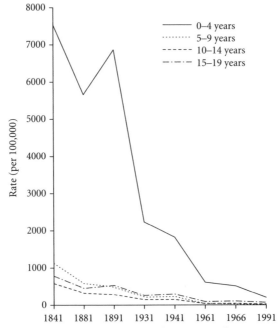

Fig. 1.2 Mortality rates in children 1841–1991. (Source: ONS.)

a part too. During the 1960s an apparently new cause of infant death appeared—sudden infant death syndrome (cot death). At the time, improved classification of deaths previously attributed to other causes (respiratory deaths or overlaying) was seen as the explanation. For two decades, sudden infant death syndrome (SIDS) became the main cause of infant death after the first month of life. Following the introduction of the 'Back to Sleep' campaign in 1991, which reversed medical advice given to parents from the 1960s onwards about the sleeping position of their baby, there was a 70% reduction in sudden infant deaths over ten years and a concomitant reduction in post-neonatal mortality rates.

The causes of death among children have also changed dramatically. Table 1.1 shows causes of death by age and sex in 1998. Accidents are now the most important cause of death after infancy. They make up 60% of all deaths at age 15–19, with an especially high rate among boys. Four per cent of deaths in the 15–19 age group are from drug abuse; this figure is likely to rise, and deaths from suicide among males in this age group are also increasing. Cancers are a significant cause of death for the 'middle years'—the 1–4, 5–9, and 10–14 age groups. There are important variations in mortality across geographical, socio-economic, and ethnic boundaries which are alluded to elsewhere in this book.

While GP consultation rates for children have remained fairly steady over the last three decades, attendance at a hospital out-patient or accident and emergency department has increased substantially—doubling in the case of 0–4 year-olds. Children aged 0–4 have an average of six GP consultations per year; those aged 5–15 have between two (boys) and three (girls). Thirteen per cent of girls and 16% of boys aged 0–4 had hospital attendances in 1998, compared to 6% and 8% respectively in 1972. The reason for the increased attendances is not fully explained. Factors which are likely to have contributed are increased expectations of healthy children amongst both parents and professionals, parental anxieties about children's illness in general, and availability of a wider range of medical interventions for both illness and disability (e.g. cancer, short stature, cystic fibrosis). Several studies suggest that there has also been a genuine increase in some common childhood health problems.

Important child health problems

Children's health problems can be grouped as follows:

- **Acute illnesses** such as otitis media, meningitis, bronchiolitis, and anaphylaxis
- **Chronic illnesses** such as asthma, epilepsy, diabetes, cancer, HIV, and AIDS
- **Disabilities** including physical and learning disabilities and sensory impairments
- **Injury**—accidental and non-accidental
- **Disorders of eating and nutrition** including failure to thrive, obesity, anorexia nervosa, and bulimia
- **Mental health disorders** such as attention deficit hyperactivity disorder (ADHD), challenging behaviour, poor sleeping, depression, anxiety, autism, and psychoses

Table 1.1 Causes of death (ICD chapter) by age and sex, Great Britain, 1998. (Source: ONS.)

Boys	28 days to under 1	1–4	5–9	10–14	15–19
All causes	2439.5	306.0	141.4	175.6	554.7
Infectious and parasitic disease (I)	188.5	31.4	7.2	4.8	17.6
Neoplasms (II)	42.2	41.6	46.0	39.4	52.8
Endocrine, nutritional, and metabolic diseases (III)	73.2	8.9	5.2	6.4	13.2
Diseases of blood and blood forming organs (IV)	14.1	4.1	2.1	1.1	2.2
Mental disorders (V)	0.0	0.0	0.0	0.0	37.9
Diseases of the nervous system and sensory organs (VI)	157.6	44.3	20.1	21.3	37.9
Diseases of the circulatory system (VII)	118.2	15.0	2.1	9.6	15.9
Diseases of the respiratory system (VIII)	261.7	29.3	9.3	8.5	15.4
Diseases of the digestive system (IX)	53.5	6.8	4.1	3.2	1.6
Diseases of the genitourinary system (X)	11.3	0.0	0.0	1.1	0.0
Diseases of the skin and subcutaneous system (XII)	0.0	0.0	0.0	0.5	0.5
Diseases of the musculoskeletal system (XIII)	0.0	0.7	1.0	1.1	1.1
Congenital anomalies (XIV)	422.1	44.3	12.4	11.2	22.5
Conditions originating in the perinatal period (XV)	472.7	6.8	0.0	0.0	0.0
Symptoms, signs, and ill-defined conditions (XVI)	517.7	12.3	1.0	0.5	6.6
Injury and poisoning (XVII)	106.9	61.4	29.9	67.1	329.3

Girls	28 days to under 1	1–4	5–9	10–14	15–19
All causes	**1953.7**	**240.6**	**111.1**	**116.7**	**266.9**
Infectious, and parasitic diseases (I)	192.4	25.9	4.9	4.5	20.3
Neoplasms (II)	23.7	30.2	30.4	16.8	34.2
Endocrine, nutritional, and metabolic diseases (III)	50.3	7.9	3.8	9.5	13.9
Diseases of blood and blood forming organs (IV)	5.9	2.2	0.5	0.6	0.6
Mental disorders (V)	2.0	1.4	0.0	1.1	9.9
Diseases of the nervous system and sense organs (VI)	127.3	30.9	20.1	23.0	23.2
Diseases of the circulatory system (VII)	88.8	20.1	6.5	5.6	13.3
Diseases of the respiratory system (VIII)	174.6	17.0	10.8	11.2	12.8
Diseases of the digestive system (IX)	47.4	5.7	2.7	2.8	3.5
Diseases of the genitourinary system (X)	5.9	1.4	0.0	0.0	0.6
Diseases of the skin and subcutaneous system (XII)	0.0	0.0	0.0	0.0	0.0
Diseases of the musculoskelatal system (XIII)	0.0	1.4	1.1	0.6	6.4
Congenital anomalies (XIV)	458.8	38.1	7.6	11.2	10.4
Conditions originating in the perinatal period (XV)	296.0	4.3	0.0	0.0	0.6
Symptoms, signs, and ill-defined conditions (XVI)	396.7	5.7	0.5	2.2	2.9
Injury and poisoning (XVII)	82.9	47.4	22.2	27.5	114.3

Acute illnesses

Acute illnesses are becoming less common and less serious as a result of immunization, better social conditions, and improved primary care. Figure 1.3 illustrates the decline in measles notifications since 1955. Progress has continued in recent years, with the introduction of both the *Haemophilus influenzae* group B (Hib) and *Neisseria meningitidis* group C (Men C) vaccines diminishing the incidence of childhood meningitis.

However, the spectre of infectious diseases has by no means been banished for good, and minor illnesses may still have a significant impact on parents and children. Expectations have changed: parents do not expect children to be ill these days and have less experience in managing illness at home, so common infectious diseases such as respiratory infections can be very worrying and the level of help sought from health professionals can be high. Partly as a result of the assumption that specific treatment is now available for all illnesses, antibiotics may be inappropriately used for some conditions, leading to increasing problems of antibiotic resistance among common pathogens and the potential for untreatable 'super bugs' in the future.

Fears about the safety of vaccines (including pertussis in the 1970s and 1980s, and MMR at the start of the current century) has led in some cases to a drop in immunization rates and to potentially serious outbreaks of whooping cough and measles. With the success of immunization in reducing death and serious morbidity, there is a tendency for the public to forget the seriousness of these diseases (there were, for example, over 250,000 deaths from measles in the UK during the twentieth century).

In addition, the emergence of new infectious diseases (most notably HIV, but also a range of others including the viral haemorrhagic fevers such as Lassa and Ebola) poses a threat worldwide which has implications for us all.

Whilst infectious diseases have generally declined in incidence and severity, the incidence of other acute conditions such as allergy and anaphylaxis has increased, creating new problems for health services and others.

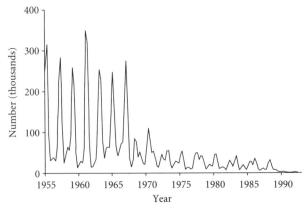

Fig. 1.3 Measles quarterly notifications: 1955–92, England and Wales. (Sources: Registrar General's Quarterly Returns 1955–73; Communicable Disease Statistics 1974–92).

Chronic illnesses

Reported rates of chronic illness in childhood more than doubled between 1972 and 1991, at a time when mortality rates continued to fall and growth rates continued to rise. This trend is continuing. This paradox may be partly explained by increasing expectations of health, greater recognition and diagnosis of certain diseases (e.g. asthma, eczema), and better survival rates of children with conditions such as cerebral palsy or cystic fibrosis due to therapeutic advances. The appearance of HIV and AIDS in the UK have posed particular challenges.

Table 1.2 Longstanding illness or disability in 0–19 year-olds for Great Britain, 2000

	2000	
	No.	%
Cancer/tumour	11	1
Diabetes	9	1
Endocrine/metabolic disorders	6	1
Mental disorders	37	4
Learning difficulties	18	2
Epilepsy	21	2
Nervous system disorders[1]	36	4
Blindness/vision defects	36	4
Deafness/ear defects	54	6
Heart disease	25	3
Diseases of the blood	8	1
Lung/respiratory disease	51	6
Asthma	373	42
Digestive disorders	37	4
Cleft palate	4	0
Urogenitary disorders	27	3
Muscoskeletal disorders	41	5
Infectious diseases	5	1
Skin conditions	72	8
Physical handicap	0	0
Other	7	1
All conditions	878	100

(Where more than one disability is present, only the main disabling condition has been included)
[1] = not elsewhere specified
Source: General Household Survey

Although increased recognition and diagnosis plays a part in inflating the apparent rise in asthma, there is evidence that there has also been a real increase, believed to be due in part to air pollution from motor vehicles and other sources. The prevalence of diabetes mellitus is also increasing, and more and more children are presenting with Type II diabetes (traditionally 'maturity onset' diabetes associated with obesity, sometimes known as 'diabesity') as well as the traditional childhood Type I or insulin-dependent diabetes.

Chronic illnesses are of great significance because of their impact on daily life. A child with chronic illness may find it difficult to participate fully in the usual pursuits of his or her age group. One of the parents (usually the mother) often has to devote a considerable amount of time to caring for the child, and her own needs may become subservient. Employment and family income may suffer, and marital relationships are often strained. Children with chronic illnesses—and those with disabilities—may require intensive services from both health and other agencies, although they and their parents usually become expert in the management of their condition.

The challenge facing those managing chronic illnesses in childhood is to balance the short term and the long term, and to take account of the child's perspective and values. Meticulous blood glucose control may carry huge benefits for the future, but if the diabetic child's life is entirely dominated by his or her condition then those benefits may be obtained at the cost of compromising the experience of childhood. Adolescents with cancer may find the side-effects of chemotherapy such an intolerable insult to their body image that they may say they would prefer not to be treated. The adults responsible for their care need to be aware of these concerns in deciding jointly what is best for the child. These patients are often amongst the most challenging for clinicians in terms of balancing the rights of children and their carers.

Disabilities

Disabilities have become a more significant aspect of child health as acute illnesses have become less common. As for chronic illnesses, quality of life is a major consideration for both parents and children. Expectations of the services and treatment available, both from health services and other agencies such as education and social services, are higher than they used to be. The demands on professionals are great, especially in the context of limited resources, and the inability to deliver the support needed by a family can be a major source of frustration.

Table 1.3 illustrates the results of a 1989 OPCS survey of childhood disability. This survey was different from previous disability surveys in that it aimed to identify the prevalence and severity of different aspects of disability rather than the medical conditions which were the underlying cause. The prevalence rates in the different categories cannot be added to give an overall prevalence of childhood disability because many children have more than one disability. The results are important, however, because they show that contrary to expectations, behavioural problems represent the most common category of functional disability. This is the case whichever level of severity of disability is considered. Problems with locomotion, continence, communication, intellectual functioning, and hearing are also significant, each with a prevalence of around one to two per hundred children.

The incidence of cerebral palsy (an important cause of disability) has increased steeply among very low birth weight babies (below 1500g), largely as a result of developments in neonatal intensive care which have led to the survival of a greater proportion of this group of babies. However, since most children born with cerebral palsy weigh over 2500g, and there has been little change in incidence among heavier babies, the overall rate has not changed significantly (Table 1.4).

The incidence of congenital anomalies has fallen dramatically with improvements in antenatal care. These include screening and termination for Down's syndrome and neural tube disorders, immunization against rubella both post-partum and in

Table 1.3 Prevalence of disability in childhood

	Per 1000
Eating/drinking/digestion	1
Disfigurement	1
Seeing	2
Reaching/stretching	2
Dexterity	4
Consciousness	5
Hearing	8
Intellectual functioning	9
Personal care	10
Locomotion	10
Communication	13
Continence	14
Behaviour	23

Source: Bone, M. and Meltzer, H. OPCS

Table 1.4 Cerebral palsy (CP) rate at different birth weights

Birth weight (g)	Perinatal mortality (per 1000 births)	Infant mortality (per 1000 births)	CP rate (per 1000 births)
<1000	525	452.4	80
1000–1499	124.1	78.6	
1500–1999	49.8	24.5	11.8
2000–2499	16.4	11.7	
2500–2999	5.4	4.2	1.26
3000–3499	2.2	2.2	

Source: Pharoah, P. et al. Arch. Dis. Child. Fetal Neonatal Ed. (1996) **75**: 169–73, with permission from the BMJ Publishing Group.

childhood, greater awareness of the teratogenic potential of certain drugs, and recommendations about folic acid intake in pregnancy. There has also been a trend towards the avoidance of foods and activities which increase the risk of infections such as listeriosis and toxoplasmosis. Overall, the number of babies born with an anomaly fell from 197 per 10,000 to 91 per 10,000 between 1986 and 1998, although part of this is due to a change in the notification system which excluded certain minor anomalies from 1991.

Accidental injury

Accidental injury continues to be the main cause of death after infancy. Although absolute rates have fallen by 25% over the last 40 years, death rates from other causes fell by nearly 75%, so that injuries represent a growing proportion of deaths among children and young people. Data gathered in the National Child Development Study cohort show that injury is now also the most common cause of physical disability in young adults.

Transport-related accidents account for one third of accidental deaths in children aged 1–4 and two-thirds in children aged 5–14. UK death and injury rates for child pedestrians are among the worst in Europe. Socio-economic inequalities in accidental death and injury rates are particularly marked: children from social class V are five times more likely to die on the roads than children in social class I. However, leisure accidents, including those due to sports, are becoming an increasingly significant cause of injury disability. Such injuries are more common among higher social classes (Fig. 1.4).

Disorders of eating and nutrition

These disorders in the UK relate mainly to inappropriate or excessive dietary intake, although certain problems of undernutrition—anorexia nervosa among adolescents and failure to thrive in infants—remain important causes of ill health in childhood.

The number of overweight and obese children continues to rise, amounting to what is now described as an obesity epidemic. Until recently, there has been no clear definition of overweight and obesity which could be used for international

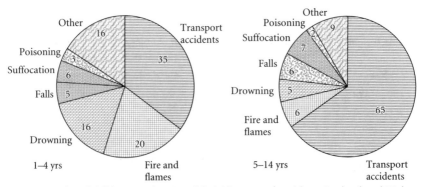

Fig. 1.4 Deaths of children aged 1–4 and 5–14 by type of accident, England and Wales, 1996–98. (Source: Mortality Statistics, Series DH2.)

comparison. The International Obesity Task Force standards have age- and gender-specific cut-offs that correspond to a BMI of 25 at age 25 years. Figures 1.5 and 1.6 show how obesity has increased in the UK, Brazil, China, Russia, and the United States.

Obesity has significant implications for health in later life as well as impacting adversely on children's peer relationships and self-esteem. Even among children of normal weight, there are concerns about the appropriateness of their diet, with many children consuming excessive amounts of saturated fat and sugar, and too little fresh fruit and vegetables and essential fatty acids such as those contained in fish oils. Dietary patterns vary between social classes, with children from more deprived backgrounds having poorer diets. Iron deficiency is prevalent in 15–40% of some child populations, particularly those from poorer backgrounds. This has consequences for child growth and brain development. The UK government's recent 'Five a Day' initiative which promotes the consumption of at least five portions of fruit and vegetables a day, and schemes to provide free fruit in schools, hope to tackle some of the problems of poor diet.

The national increase in the incidence of food poisoning is also relevant, especially to younger and immunocompromised children who are at greater risk of serious illness from infections such as *E. coli 0157*.

Eating disorders such as anorexia nervosa and bulimia are an increasing problem especially among adolescent girls. Such girls are highly subject to media images of underweight women appearing as fashion models, and also to peer influence which can generate 'outbreaks' in schools.

There has been an improvement in dental health which owes a great deal to the addition of fluoride to toothpaste and drinking water, but there are now marked socio-economic and regional variations related to the inequitable geographic distribution of water fluoridation as well as to high sugar consumption. A very large proportion of dental caries in the child population, clusters in a small proportion of children from deprived backgrounds. Although dental care is available free on the NHS to children, in some areas NHS dentists are hard to find.

Breast-feeding confers health advantages to the infant, the developing child, and the young adult—as well as to the mother (see box below).

Advantages of breast-feeding

For the baby	For the mother
Lower risk of gastrointestinal infections	Cheap
Lower risk of respiratory infections	Convenient – no sterilizing or bottle
Lower risk of atopic disorders	preparation
Possibly, higher IQ in preterms	No risk of error in composition
Lower risk of cot death	Promotes post-partum weight loss
Lower risk of heart disease in later life	Lower risk of breast cancer
	May promote mother-infant relationship

Breast-feeding rates have improved over the last two or three decades but the increase has been slow in recent years, from a total of 66% at birth in 1995 to 69%

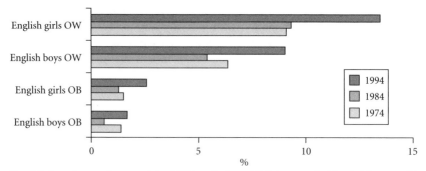

Fig. 1.5 Prevalence of overweight (OW) and obese (OB) boys and girls, 4–11 years old, 1974–94. (Source: Chinn and Rona *BMJ* (2001) **322**: 24–6, with permission from the BMJ Publishing Group.)

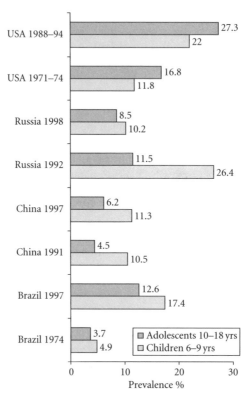

Fig. 1.6 Trends in obesity prevalence in USA, Russia, China, and Brazil. (Source: Wang, Y. *et al.* (2002). *Am. J. Clin. Nutrition*; **75**: 971–7. Permission sought.)

in 2000. The numbers maintaining breast-feeding are even lower: there is a sharp and continuing decline over the first few weeks and months, so that only one in five mothers are still breast-feeding at six months. The incidence of breast-feeding is higher for first babies than subsequent births, and there are significant differences between social and ethnic groups. The majority of mothers in social class I breast-feed, compared to relatively small numbers in social class V, although figures from 2000 show a narrowing of this gap. Breast-feeding rates among mothers from the Asian subcontinent and of African or Caribbean origin are substantially higher than among white mothers. There have been improvements in hospital and community support with the development of the UNICEF Baby Friendly Award (see Chapter 7), but these are slow to influence breast-feeding rates.

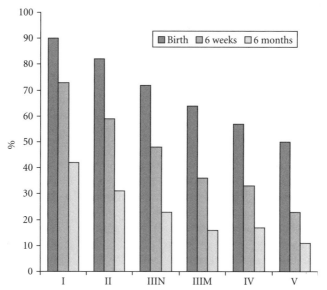

Fig. 1.7 Breast-feeding rates by social class (birth, 6 weeks, and 6 months) in Great Britain. (Source: 1995 ONS.)

Table 1.5 Incidence of breast-feeding by birth order and ethnic group

	% breast-feeding initially			
	Bangladeshi	**Pakistani**	**Indian**	**White**
First birth	94	80	89	72
Second and subsequent births	88	74	77	54

Source: 1995 ONS

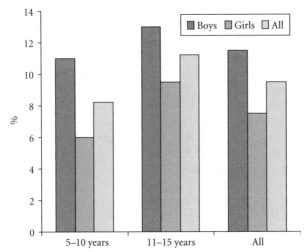

Fig. 1.8 Prevalence of mental health disorders in children (Source: *Mental health of children and adolescents in Great Britain*, ONS, 2001).

Mental health disorders

Mental health disorders are increasingly prevalent at all ages. Data on prevalence depend on diagnostic criteria, which may vary from study to study. However, it is estimated that approximately one in ten children over the age of five have a significant mental health disorder. A large survey of children in Great Britain demonstrated that in the age group 5–15 years, 5% had clinically significant conduct disorders, 4% were assessed as having emotional disorders (anxiety and depression), and 1% were hyperactive (Fig. 1.8).

The diagnosis of attention deficit hyperactivity disorder (ADHD) is rising, though this may be due as much to improved recognition as to changes in occurrence. Conduct disorder is also thought to be increasing in prevalence. Behavioural problems in general pose challenges to all services for children (health, mental health, educational, and social services) and place a particular burden on already stressed teachers. Reasons for the increase may include the widening gap between rich and poor, changing parenting styles, increasing rates of teenage parenthood, and more single parenthood, all of which impact adversely on children's mental health.

Depression and anxiety among children and young people is also increasing, as are rates of parasuicide and deliberate self-harm. In England and Wales the suicide rate for young men aged 15–19 years has climbed steadily since the mid 1970s. This may be related to increases in divorce and unemployment.

The diagnosis of autism and Asperger's syndrome continues to rise steadily, placing great strain on the specialist services needed to provide for these children, especially the early intervention services which offer some hope of better integration in the medium term.

Summary

The reduction in mortality and morbidity from infectious disease has been replaced by new 'morbidities of modern living' which affect the children of most developed countries. Many of the areas of concern are outlined above and include a rise in mental ill health and developmental disorders, injury, obesity, and the health effects of poverty. These are some of the challenges facing child public health professionals at the beginning of the twenty-first century.

The determinants of health in children

A wide range of factors influence the health of both children and adults. These can be represented in diagrammatic terms as a series of concentric circles radiating out from the individual through his or her immediate social environment and circumstances (the family and local community) to society as a whole and the wider socioeconomic and physical environment. The Mandala diagram has been used for centuries to describe this idea (see Fig. 1.9).

The second half of this chapter will explore the major determinants of health in children in the UK, setting the scene for instigating action to improve child health later in the book.

Key determinants of health in children

- Poverty and income inequality
- Families and relationships
- Nutrition
- The physical and social environment
- Social attitudes and stigma
- Risk behaviour
- Genetics
- Health service provision

Poverty and income inequality

Poverty is a key factor influencing health worldwide. Children are more affected by socio-economic circumstances than any other age group in society. There is a strong school of thought that, in the affluent developed world, where famine and drought are now more or less unheard of, it is *relative* rather than *absolute* poverty which is critical. Others believe it is absolute levels of poverty that matter. The distinction is important because the effects of absolute poverty can be mitigated or abolished by increasing the income and resources available to the very poor. The effects of relative poverty, however, cannot be solved without redistributing income—reducing the income of the rich at the same time as increasing the income of the poor.

Those contributing to the child public health literature in European Union (EU) countries usually base their research on relative measures of poverty, the most common of which assesses the proportion of households with incomes less than 50% of the national average. Chapter 4 discusses different methods of measuring poverty and income inequality in more detail, including comparative and subjective measures.

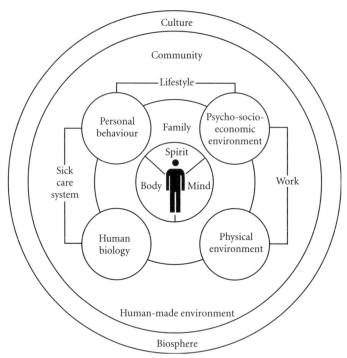

Fig. 1.9 The Mandala diagram of health—a model of the human ecosystem. (Source: Hancock, T. (1985). Family and Community Health **8**: 1–10.)

Poverty in the UK

Using the EU definition, the UK does not compare well with other industrialized countries with regard to the extent of child poverty: the level of inequality between rich and poor in this country has been rising steadily for the last 20 years. Figure 1.10 shows the percentage of children living below national poverty lines.

Overall, of 47 million children in the 29 rich countries of the Organization for Economic Cooperation and Development (OECD), one in six lives below nationally defined poverty lines. Whilst child poverty remained stable or increased only slightly across most OECD countries in the last 20 years, it tripled in Britain. The UK is fourth from the bottom with 19.8% in relative poverty, and USA second bottom with 22.5%. Child poverty in Britain is twice as high as in France and five times higher than Norway or Sweden (see Figs. 1.10, 1.11).

There are three main reasons for the increase in child poverty in the UK in recent years:

1. Unemployment

2. An increase in the number of lone-parent families

3. Changes in the tax and benefits system. Townsend (in *Inequalities in health* (Gordon, D. *et al.*)) identifies as particularly significant the abolition of the link between social security benefits and earnings, the restraints on the value of Child Benefit, the abolition of lone-parent allowances and of the earnings-related

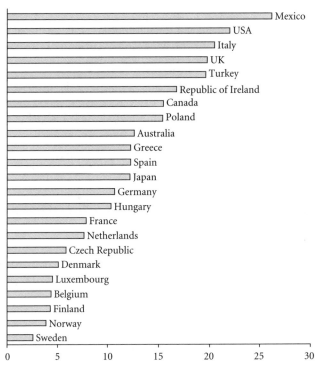

Fig. 1.10 Percentage of children living in 'relative' poverty (households with income below 50% of national median). (Source: Innocenti Research Centre *BMJ* (2000) **320**: 1621, with permission from the BMJ Publishing Group.)

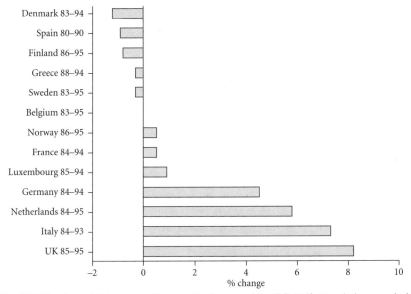

Fig. 1.11 Trends in child poverty. (Source: Bradbury and Jantii (1999). Permission sought.)

addition to Incapacity Benefit, and the substitution of means-tested benefits for universal social insurance and non-contributory benefits for certain groups.

The impact of poverty on child health

The profound effects of socio-economic circumstances on children's health are eloquently demonstrated by the social class differences in childhood mortality illustrated opposite. Although the impact on mortality is most marked in the poorest groups, there is a clear trend across all social groups, suggesting that both absolute and relative poverty are important. If absolute poverty were the only problem, we would expect to see increased mortality only in the poorest groups, whereas the trend across all social classes suggests an effect of relative poverty.

Social class differentials in mortality rates are most marked for child pedestrian accidents and deaths from fires, but there is no main cause of death for which children in lower social classes have lower rates than children in higher classes. A northern region study of deaths involving head injuries showed a 15-fold difference in mortality between the most deprived and the least deprived deciles of local authority electoral wards. Social class effects are also evident in the rates of congenital malformations and chronic illness.

Poverty, income inequality, and variations in health

The Black Report, published in 1980, was important in bringing the issue of social inequalities in health back onto the public health agenda (see Chapter 3 for discussion about poverty and health in earlier times). This report, which covered inequalities from cradle to grave, discussed four of the explanations for variations in health across social classes which have been put forward:

1. an artefact of the measurement process

2. natural selection (lower social classes are inevitably made up of weaker people who cannot improve their circumstances)

3. structural problems (poverty and social deprivation affect health adversely)

4. cultural/behavioural ('people harm themselves by the excessive consumption of harmful commodities').

The authors presented data which enabled them to discount the first explanation. The second argument, remarkable as it may seem to readers in the twenty-first century, used to inform public health policy in the past (see Chapter 3) but is no longer accepted as a valid argument. The fourth explanation was the one favoured by the Conservative government of the day, but several careful studies have since concluded that differences in health-related lifestyles are insufficient to account for social inequalities in health. Such differences are also now recognized to be heavily influenced by structural factors, since individuals' socio-economic circumstances have a profound effect on the choices open to them. The authors of the Black Report concluded that the wider issues of class differentials and their impact on living circumstances (structural issues) were the fundamental cause. They did not explicitly touch on the debate about the relative importance of absolute and relative poverty.

The arguments in favour of the importance of relative poverty are well described by Wilkinson (1992). He discusses three interpretations which might be put on data

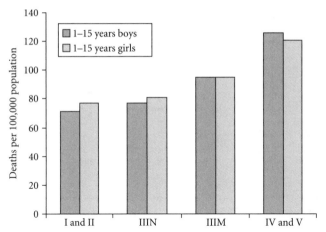

Fig. 1.12 Mortality (all causes) of children 1–15 years by sex and social class (1983). (Source: ONS.)

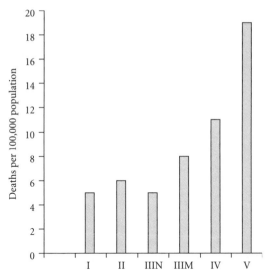

Fig. 1.13 Mortality from injury in children aged 1–14 years, by social class, 1982–3. (Source: ONS.)

showing that countries with wider income disparities have poorer health:

1. the individual income interpretation
2. the neo-material interpretation
3. the psychosocial environment interpretation.

The first suggests that the association between income inequality and health at population level merely reflects the aggregated association at individual level—an

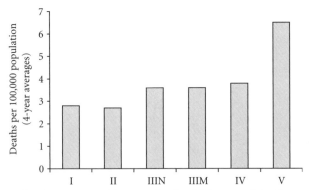

Fig. 1.14 Mortality from congential anomalies in children aged 1–14 years, by social class, 1979–83. (Source: ONS.)

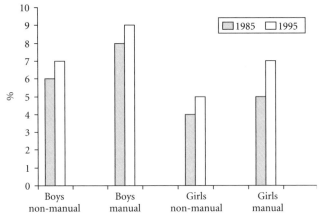

Fig. 1.15 Prevalence of reported limiting longstanding illlness in children under 16 years in Great Britain, 1985 and 1995. (Source: ONS.)

argument compatible with the absolute poverty approach. Several studies have, however, shown that national patterns of income distribution have health effects which remain after adjustment for individual income levels within the country, so although individual income is important, something else must explain the observed relationships between income inequality and health.

The neo-material interpretation (favoured by the Black Report) states that health problems among those with low incomes are simply due to lack of provision—of education, health services, transportation, food, housing, and so on. This interpretation is also compatible with an absolute poverty explanation, and remedies for it do not need to involve income redistribution. Improving access to high-quality services and housing should have a beneficial effect.

The psychosocial environment interpretation provides a possible explanation of the mechanisms involved in the impact of relative poverty. It proposes that psychosocial factors are vital in mediating the effect of income inequalities. Those at the lower end of the social scale feel marginalized and excluded, self-esteem suffers, and feelings of powerlessness (both real and imagined) impede lifestyle and environmental change. The distress induced by powerlessness and poor self-esteem may lead to poorer health via a variety of physiological mechanisms which are being explored through research in psychoneuroimmunology. These might include hypertension, lowered immune response, and abnormal clotting mechanisms. If this explanation were the most important, remedies which mitigate the effects of poverty by, for example, providing better education or health services for the poor, would not solve the problem on their own. Redistributive policies which reduce the gap in wealth between rich and poor would be essential. Measures to improve social cohesion might also be helpful, since social cohesion at community level could be expected to mitigate some of these psychosocial effects (see discussion of social capital in Chapter 4).

The priorities for public health action to address the impact of income inequality clearly depend on the interpretation which is favoured. It is likely that all three contribute, but the exact balance is unclear. Broad based action is indicated, focussing on obtaining a more equitable distribution of public and private resources, improving social cohesion, and improving service provision and structural barriers to health.

How does poverty affect children's health in practice?

It follows from the arguments above that several mechanisms are likely to be involved in mediating the influence of socio-economic circumstances on children's health, not all of them directly related to lack of money. They include:

- **the direct effects of low income** e.g. insufficient or inappropriate food, lack of heating, and damp housing
- **the environmental effects of living in a poor neighbourhood** e.g. lack of safe play areas and leisure facilities, poor schools
- **the psychosocial effects of poverty** e.g. low self-esteem, powerlessness, parental stress precipitating family conflict and domestic violence, parental drug and alcohol abuse, inadequate supervision, parental depression, crime, violence, and lack of social capital in communities (see Chapter 4).

The box below illustrates some of these mechanisms.

Poverty and child health: some examples

Accidents Accidents to children in the home are strongly influenced by the environment, which is in its turn affected by poverty. Falls and burns are more likely to occur in houses not designed with safety in mind and in the absence of safety equipment such as smoke detectors, stairgates, fireguards, and cooker guards. Safety equipment is expensive and not always easy to obtain, and low-income families are more likely to live in houses that are unsafe, overcrowded, and have old electrical equipment. Motor vehicle accidents are more likely if children have to play in the street. Children may be less well supervised in lone-parent families or where parents both work or have health problems of their own; and older siblings may have to look after younger ones at an

Effects of poverty on children's health

Factor	Effect on health
Insufficient or inappropriate food	Undernutrition, malnutrition, obesity
Damp and cold housing	Respiratory infections
Small, overcrowded housing	Increased infection risk
Lack of play space in garden or locally	Increased accident risk (especially road traffic accidents)
Low self-esteem and powerlessness	Difficulty making supportive relationships and lifestyle changes
Parental stress and conflict	Behaviour problems; increased risk of child abuse
Lack of stimulation and play	Poor educational achievement
Lack of supervision	Increased accident risk; behaviour problems
Lack of social capital; crime; violence	Anxiety; bullying; drug abuse; parental illness

earlier age than is appropriate. Environmental modification and better provision for children's play is essential if accidental injuries are to be reduced in low-income areas.

Teenage pregnancy The strong links between teenage pregnancy and low income, as well as other indicators of deprivation, were recognized in the allocation of governmental responsibility for teenage pregnancy in the UK to the government's Social Exclusion Unit. Girls under 16 from deprived areas were shown in a Scottish study to be three times more likely to become pregnant than those from privileged areas, but less likely to have the pregnancy terminated. Overall, rates of teenage pregnancy are up to ten times higher in social class V than social class I. Teenage mothers are six times more likely to have no qualifications than the general population; 'Looked After' children (children in public care) are at greater risk of becoming teenage parents; and one in three male young offenders are fathers. This illustrates the tendency of factors associated with deprivation and poor health to 'cluster'—and since teenage pregnancy itself is a cause of poorer health in both the teenage mother and her baby, it perpetuates inequalities through generations.

Possible explanations for the high rate of pregnancy among poorer and deprived teenagers include educational failure and lack of career opportunities, low self-esteem, and the perceived opportunities for independent living resulting from motherhood.

Families, family structure, parent–child relationships, and parenting

Family structure

The family provides a child's immediate social network: family structure and function is therefore a vital influence on children's health and well-being. As a result of changing gender attitudes and expectations, marital breakdown is now more common than ever before (40% of first marriages end in divorce) and single-parent families are on the increase.

Reconstituted families are also much more common. Many children experience the presence of a step-parent and step-siblings and their care may be shared between parents who do not live together. If it is possible for parents or others to continue to provide loving care and security then children's emotional and social development may not suffer, but clearly there is a greater vulnerability when conflict between parents is common.

Family break-up and conflict

It is not unusual for children's health and well-being to suffer from family breakdown. Emotional and behavioural problems and educational failure are more common, and children in these circumstances are also more likely to be abused. Some have suggested that it is not the single-parent family status or the family breakdown themselves which are the problem, but the poverty which often accompanies these situations. Others have suggested that what damages children is exposure to conflict. Persistent unresolved conflict in the home is detrimental to children's social and emotional development. Children who grow up in homes characterized by marital discord, particularly where there is verbal or physical aggression, non-verbal conflict, or the 'silent treatment,' are at increased risk of emotional and behavioural problems. Sometimes children, particularly girls, may respond to conflict by adopting a parental role themselves. All these outcomes put children at increased risk of experiencing mental health problems and difficulty in establishing healthy relationships in later life. Persistent unresolved conflict, including domestic violence, occurs in all social classes.

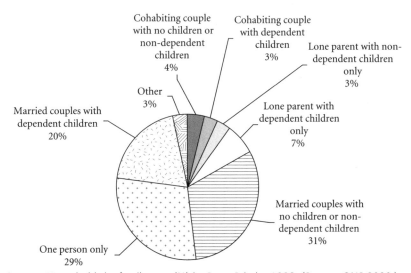

Fig. 1.16 Households by family type (%) in Great Britain, 1998. (Source: ONS 2000.)

Early parent–child relationships

From the moment of birth, the way mothers and fathers relate to their babies has an important influence on their emotional and social development. The mother–child relationship can be measured, at one year of age, by the observed responses of the baby to temporary separation. The degree of 'attachment' predicts the following in later years:

◆ self-confidence
◆ self-efficacy
◆ self-regulation
◆ autonomy
◆ good relationships with peers.

Adolescents who were securely attached at age one are more competent, more socially orientated and empathetic, more able to develop deeper relationships, and more likely to respond to stress by seeking help than those who were insecurely attached at this age.

Babies develop in response to social interaction and are active players in the relationship. The baby's temperament plays a part in this process, and some babies are

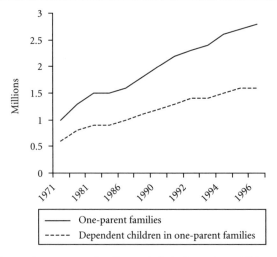

Health effects of family break-up and domestic violence

◆ Emotional and behavioural problems
◆ Poor personal relationships and difficulty in dealing with conflict
◆ Increased risk of child abuse
◆ Poverty
◆ Increased likelihood of violence in the children

Fig. 1.17 Numbers of one-parent families and their dependent children, Great Britain, 1971–96. (Source: ONS 2000.)

more difficult to soothe than others. However, the babies of mothers who are not able to 'read' their infants and are not in tune with their needs become anxious and withdrawn. In the longer term, these babies fail to develop the self-soothing mechanisms that older children and adults depend on to respond helpfully to stress. Children who are insecurely attached at one year of age are likely to be anxious, aggressive, or isolated at school. Babies who are nurtured in a way sensitive to their needs seem to be able to weather the adverse consequences of living in poverty and deprivation, emerging unscathed into adulthood. Thus, secure attachment supports the development of resilience and insecure attachment creates vulnerability to psychopathology in later life.

There are strong intergenerational links in attachment styles, so parents tend to parent their children in the way that they themselves were parented. Post-natal depression

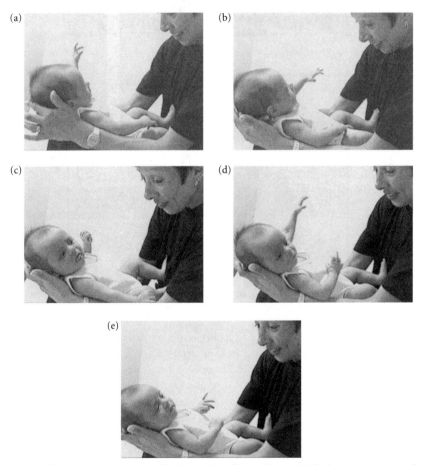

Fig. 1.18 How parents can 'read' their baby (from *The social baby* Murray, L. and Andrews, E. (ed.) The Children's Project www.socialbaby.com <http://www.socialbaby.com>). Alexandra shows that she is tiring of the conversation (c), by turning her head away and watching her mother from the corner of her eye. Then she cuts her gaze completely (d). In (e), she is recharged and shows that she is ready for further conversation.

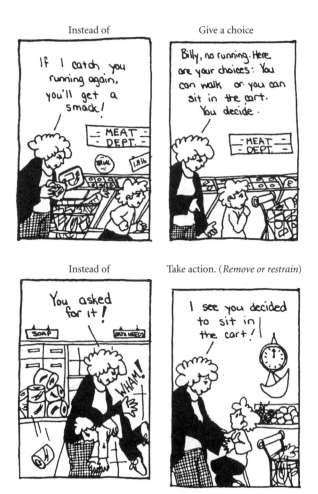

Fig. 1.19 An illustration of positive discipline. From Faber, A., Mazlish, E. (1980) How to talk so kids will listen and listen so kids will talk. Avon Books, New York. Permission sought.

is an interrupter of attachment, and babies whose mothers have been depressed are more likely to demonstrate difficulties in adjustment to school, difficulties in relating to peers, and emotional and behavioural problems typical of insecurely attached children. Problems with attachment are more common amongst mothers living in social deprivation, and many intervention studies have concentrated on trying to improve attachment in this group. There are now a number of psychotherapeutically based interventions which have been shown to help the mothers of insecurely attached infants become more in tune with their babies. These are collectively referred to as interventions which promote infant mental health (see Chapter 7). Those working in this field are increasingly aware that it is not just the relationship with the mother that counts: attachment to fathers is also important. Interventions to support fathering are beginning to be developed, but the evidence base for these is not yet well established.

Parent–child relationships in childhood and adolescence

Later in childhood, boundaries become an issue of importance for social and emotional development and mental health. Harsh and inconsistent discipline, poor monitoring and supervision, and lack of warmth, affection, and praise are all important determinants of antisocial behaviour and conduct disorder in children, and delinquency, violence, and criminality in adolescence. Paterson and his colleagues at the Oregon Social Learning Centre have shown that these parenting styles alone account for as much as 40% of the variation in conduct disorder.

A useful classification, which owes its origins to Diana Baumrind, describes parenting styles as:

- **authoritative**—loving and understanding, with firm, age-appropriate, and negotiated boundaries
- **authoritarian**—punitive and unaffectionate
- **neglectful**—neither loving nor firm
- **permissive**—loving, but failing to exercise any control.

Children of parents who are authoritative do much better at school, have higher self-esteem, and more rewarding peer interactions than those whose parents adopt other styles.

Another approach to the classification of parenting distinguishes between just two different dimensions of parenting—support and control. This classification emphasizes the positive aspects of parental support and the negative aspects of intrusive parental control. Overcontrolling parenting styles can have a negative impact on the development of autonomy. Children of parents who are controlling and unsupportive are most at risk of unhealthy lifestyles and poor educational outcomes. Good communication with parents in adolescence, which is unlikely to feature in families where parents are controlling or unsupportive, can protect against the adoption of unhealthy lifestyles.

A large number of interventions have been developed to help parents of children between 2 and 11 years change the way they parent and, as we shall see in Chapter 7, the evidence base for some of these interventions is impressive.

Abuse and neglect

Child abuse and neglect represent the extreme end of the continuum of unhelpful parenting. Abuse may be physical, emotional, or sexual, or take the form of neglect or failure to thrive. Abuse can occur in families from all social classes, although physical abuse and neglect (but not sexual abuse) are more common in manual class families. It is most common when the parents themselves were abused as children, among parents who abuse alcohol or drugs or who have mental health problems, and when the child has a disability. Abuse or neglect have profound effects on children's physical and mental health, often leading to failure to thrive, to repeated injuries, to withdrawal, mental illness, and emotional and behavioural problems—and to abusive relationships with partners and children in later life. The most serious cases can be fatal: one or two children a week die at the hands of their parents or carers in the UK, although the NSPCC believes this to be a significant underestimate.

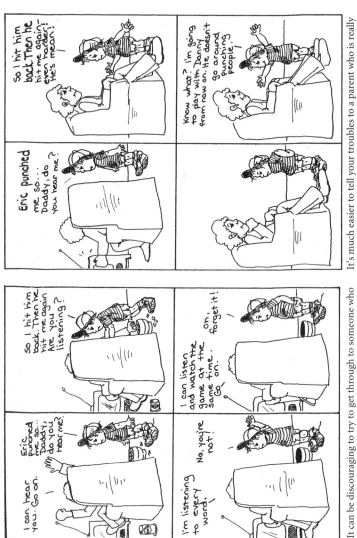

Fig. 1.20 The effect of listening well (from Faber and Mazlich). Permission sought.

Discipline

The boundary between abuse and acceptable punishment is not clearly defined and is changing with time. The acceptability of any form of physical punishment in particular is now questionable. Several studies have shown that while physical punishment may interrupt problem behaviour and relieve parental frustration, in the longer term it increases rather than reduces antisocial behaviour. Any form of physical punishment is an assault and models the belief that it is acceptable for the powerful to control the powerless by force. It is also in clear breach of the UN Convention on the Rights of the Child. Some European countries now regard physical punishment as abusive and have brought in legislation to protect children from physical discipline.

Nutrition

Poor nutrition is related to the cost and availability of healthy food and the convenience of unhealthy food, to parents' experience of and available time for cooking, and to cultural attitudes, which may be heavily influenced by intensive media marketing of high-calorie, high-sugar, and low-fibre foods. It is hard for parents to control food quality as few families grow their own food. Most buy it in the supermarket, and the basis of their choice is often marketing (much of it aimed at children) rather than nutritional principles. Several surveys have shown that a 'healthy' food basket (containing fruit, vegetables, and fish, for example) is considerably more expensive than an 'unhealthy' basket (containing food such as pies, chips, and sausages). This difference is more marked in inner city estates lacking markets where good-quality vegetables can be purchased cheaply, and in low-income families without a car who are unable to 'shop around' for bargains.

When a higher proportion of the household budget goes on food, adults are reluctant to buy food that might be thrown away if the children do not like it. Thus children's preferences, influenced by advertising, may affect the family diet unduly. Families from ethnic minorities who find it hard to access culturally appropriate ingredients may well fall back on the most familiar and least healthy options among the 'traditional' UK diet.

Nutritional awareness in the community is low and labelling information can be abstruse and confusing. Cooking facilities may be limited; parents may lack culinary skills or education and have little experience of eating a variety of foods. Food additives are ubiquitous, especially in soft drinks and the convenience foods that are attractive to children; these may lead to hyperactivity and to migraine as well as being possibly addictive. There is also a high content of 'hidden' salt and sugar in many products.

The effects of marketing, children's preferences, cost, and the composition of many convenience foods thus lead to a skewing of the diet, especially in low-income families, towards high saturated fat, high salt, high sugar, and low fibre intake. The detrimental health effects of such a diet include higher risks of coronary heart disease, cancer, obesity, and dental caries. Currently, 20% of children eat no fruit. It has been estimated that increasing fruit and vegetable intake to five pieces a day across the population is potentially the second most effective strategy for reducing cancer after curbing smoking, and could reduce deaths from chronic disease overall by 20%. Health education alone cannot change the situation: initiatives such as food co-operatives, farmer's markets in cities, and the government's National School Fruit Scheme can make an important contribution.

Education

A large number of studies have shown education to be an important determinant of health. High-quality preschool provision, particularly when combined with parenting education and support, can combat some of the health problems associated with social inequalities. Later, high educational achievement makes secure, well-paid employment more likely and sets the foundation for the lifelong learning which supports health and personal development.

Environment

Their physical and social environment has a major impact on children's life and health. Poor air quality is common in large cities as a result of traffic and industrial emissions and can exacerbate or precipitate respiratory disorders. Housing quality is variable and in disadvantaged areas is associated with dampness, poor heating, and overcrowding. Public transport may be poor or non-existent, with the result that children have to be transported by car or walk long distances. Lack of good public transport makes it difficult for children from low-income families to get to leisure centres and the countryside (important environments for children's health and well-being). In inner city areas there is often inadequate safe play space, so that children either play in the streets or are kept in the house because of parents' fears for their safety.

Television

The influence of television is pervasive and often negative. Children are less often allowed to play outside as a result of parental anxiety, and because of the popularity of television as a source of entertainment (as well as a resident 'babysitter' for busy parents), many spend increasing hours in front of a screen either watching television or videos, on the internet, or playing interactive games. In the USA, 9–10 year-old children watch about 15.5 hours of television and 5 hours of videos every week, and play 3 hours of video games. This carries direct health costs as well as opportunity

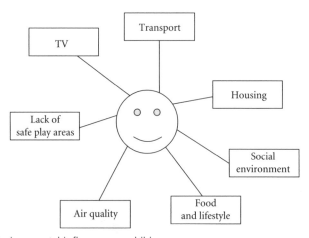

Fig. 1.21 Environmental influences on children.

costs. The direct costs come from exposure to the marketing of unhealthy food and drink, to the influence of violence, sexual permissiveness, and alcohol abuse, and to a predominance of male gender values. The opportunity costs are a reduction in physical activity, interactive family life, and conversation, the latter being especially adverse in young children during the period of language acquisition.

Claims have been made for the educational value of television watching, but they depend on the involvement of active learning, which is rare: television watching is essentially a passive activity. If parents discuss programmes with children after watching together, the benefit is said to be increased, but the extent to which this happens is not known.

Television: good or bad for children?

Beneficial effects of TV	Adverse effects of TV
Reduced stress on parents	Delays language development
Potential educational benefit	Modelling of violence
Shared family activity	Advertising of junk food
	Reduced activity levels
	Reduced family interaction
	Modelling of sexual activity

Recent research has shown that reducing the amount of time that primary school children spend watching television and playing video games can make them less aggressive towards their peers, making this an important area for parent and professional education. Reducing television watching has also been shown to contribute to weight loss in overweight children. However, since television is now an integral part of society any public health approach to protect children must be tempered with realism and recognize the importance of market forces. Possible means of controlling the adverse effects of TV on children are shown in the box.

Television: how to curtail its adverse influence on children

- Public education (e.g. American Academy of Pediatrics 'Media Matters' Campaign, see *www.aap.org*)
- School education on media literacy
- Paediatrician education (as above, not yet evaluated)
- TV 'limiter' (allows parents to control internet use)
- State control of media violence
- Legislation to curb advertising of junk foods to children

Social environment

Children's social environment also affects their health. Important factors include social isolation, fear of crime, and lack of social support in the community at large. These are discussed in more detail in Chapter 4 in the section on social capital. The school environment is also important. School ethos has been shown to have a profound effect on children's mental health and self-esteem. Many children do not feel safe at school and anxiety is an important inhibitor of learning. The extent to which children are treated with respect at school is important for the development of autonomy. A caring environment and zero tolerance of emotional or physical bullying is important. One of the key factors in determining school ethos is the emotional and social well-being of staff, and current school health promotion programmes (e.g. the national Healthy Schools Scheme) includes improving staff mental health as one of its goals. These schemes take a universal approach, covering the physical and social environment of the school, relationships with parents and the wider community, and class-based activities.

Summary

The health effects of the environment are summarized in the box.

Health effects of the environment

Poor air quality	→	respiratory disease
Poor housing	→	asthma, respiratory infections
Excessive use of cars	→	accidents, lack of exercise, obesity
No safe play areas	→	accidents on the street, lack of exercise, obesity
Television	→	obesity, delayed language, violence
Social isolation	→	fear of crime, lack of social support
School ethos	→	positive or negative effect on emotional well-being and behaviour

---

Social attitudes and stigma

Attitudes to children and parents in society

It is often said that the UK is not a child-centred society. The examples cited usually relate to negative public attitudes to children and parents, and to negative coverage of children in the media (e.g. the focus on child crime and truancy). Familiar anecdotal evidence includes the lack of welcome given to children in restaurants and other public places compared to other European countries, negative images of teenagers in the street, disapproval of and lack of facilities for breast-feeding in public places, and the low importance and priority UK society accords to parenting (for full-time mothers, but especially full-time fathers). Perhaps more important is the presence or absence of legislation to protect children and promote their well-being. The box below gives examples of positive and negative aspects of legislation and planning in the UK. While we are doing well in some areas, we have some way to go to match our Scandinavian neighbours in recognizing and valuing the contribution of children to our society.

Intolerance and stigma

Social exclusion is a feature of society in all westernized countries and profoundly affects children's health. Social exclusion means the handicap imposed on an individual or group as a result of their position in society: it may result from poverty, behaviour, mental health problems, race or religion, gender, or sexual orientation.

Are children protected and supported by government in the UK?

Yes	No
• Child labour laws	• Physical punishment still legal
• Compulsory education	• Lack of universally available child care
• Child protection legislation	• Limited maternity leave
• Children Act (England)	• Very limited paternity leave
• Child Benefit	• No Children's Rights Commissioner in England**
• Universal health visitor service	• Few facilities for adolescents in NHS
• UK has ratified UN Convention on Children's Rights (but excluded asylum seekers)	• No consultation with children on policy matters (but government is committed to improving this)
• New Minister for Children and the Family (2003)	

**Commissioners are proposed in Wales, Scotland, and Northern Ireland

Several groups of children may suffer from the negative effects of intolerance and stigma. These include the poor, those from minority ethnic groups, asylum seekers, travellers, disabled children, and 'Looked-After' children.

Ethnicity and culture Life is difficult for many ethnic minority children in the UK. The problems they face include a higher prevalence of poverty (often exacerbated by poverty in the home country and discrimination that reduces job prospects in the UK), racist attitudes, and bullying at school (especially for those for whom English is a second language). In some cases there are difficulties of acculturation (for example, cultural differences in expectation compared to the UK norm, especially for girls in Islamic families, and a lack of continuity in contact with services among traveller families). These collectively confer both physical and mental health risks. For children of asylum seekers, the experience of war, torture, human rights abuses, and flight, often compounded by the loss of close family members, can leave deep psychological scars; many arrive in this country unaccompanied by family or friends. It is vital that professionals are aware of all these issues and provide culturally appropriate care and services for all such children, using interpreters when needed.

Disability Although there have been improvements in recent years, there is still discrimination against people with a disability, and access is a vital part of this. How easy is it for a child in a wheelchair to get around the school, to take a bus or train, or to go shopping in town?

The inclusion of children with disabilities in mainstream schools is potentially beneficial both for them and for the wider school population, leading to greater integration and better understanding and social acceptance of disability. However, there is also the potential for failing to meet such children's educational and social needs: if there is insufficient support in the school then bullying and isolation are common. This is particularly so for children with learning difficulties, when there are no outward signs to explain why the child is struggling or needs extra help.

Risk behaviour and adolescent health

During preadolescence and adolescence, children adopt health-related lifestyles which together play a part in the maintenance of health and contribute to the development of the diseases which cause morbidity and premature mortality in adulthood. Diet and nutrition and exercise participation are key elements, as are high-risk behaviours such as substance use and misuse (smoking, alcohol, mood altering drugs) and unsafe sex. During infancy and early childhood, parental lifestyles not only have an important direct impact on child health (for example, the effects of smoking, alcohol, and drug misuse, and lack of breast-feeding) but also provide negative models for children. These parental behaviour patterns are all more common amongst families living in poverty. Access to high-quality, culturally appropriate food is also closely linked with poverty, as we have already seen, and opportunities for exercise may depend on the availability of play areas and leisure facilities.

Experimenting with unhealthy lifestyles is common in young people from all social backgrounds, but children from more deprived backgrounds are more likely to continue these behavioural patterns into adulthood. High-risk behaviour among teenagers is on the increase because of greater affluence at this age, more independence, and the marketing of drugs, alcohol, and sex in the media. The UK has the highest rate of teenage pregnancy in Europe and epidemic levels of sexually transmitted infections. Binge alcohol drinking is also among the highest in Europe among young people and 29% of 15-year-old girls are regular smokers (*Child Health Statistics 2000*). Smoking among 16–19 year-olds has declined less than in the population as a whole. Deaths among children and teenagers from volatile substance abuse rose steeply between 1980 and 1990 to a figure of around 100 per year, and 26% of 15-year-old boys reported using an illicit drug in a 1998 survey (see Figs. 1.22 and 1.23 opposite).

Genetics

Genetic predisposition plays a part in determining the health of children. For a small number, specific genetic defects lead directly to specific conditions such as cystic fibrosis, Down's syndrome, or haemophilia. Children from certain ethnic backgrounds are at greater risk of particular genetic diseases such as thalassaemia and sickle cell anaemia. Consanguinity increases the risk of particular conditions among groups for whom this is a common cultural practice. It is important that health professionals are aware of these risks and alert to the possibility of rare diseases, so that they can offer appropriate care and counselling. The rapid rise in understanding of genetic conditions offers the potential for intervention and also for screening, either antenatally or post-natally or sometimes in later childhood; it also raises complex ethical issues which society needs to address. In the future, genetic manipulation may make it easier for parents to choose to remove defects in their unborn infant. It will be important for health service providers to ensure that information is available to parents of all backgrounds and education.

Health service provision

The perceived importance of health service provision as a determinant of health has waxed and waned. For a period in the latter half of the twentieth century, following the foundation of the NHS, it was seen as the single most important factor affecting the health of the population; more recently, growing awareness of the role of social and environmental determinants of health led to a swing in the opposite direction, with health services seen by many as a minor player in public health terms.

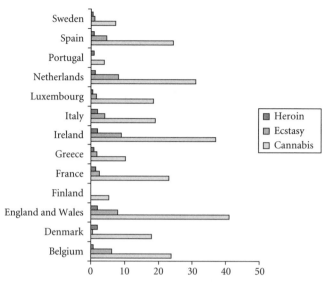

Fig. 1.22 Lifetime prevalence (%) of use of different illegal drugs among 15–16 year-old students. (Source: *EC Report on the State of Young People's Health in the European Union* (2000).)

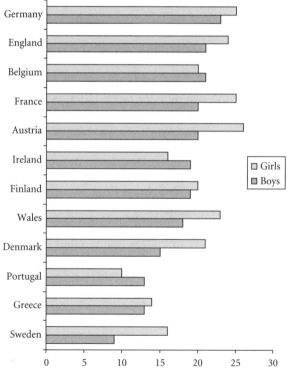

Fig. 1.23 Percentages of 15-year-olds who report smoking daily. (Source: *EC Report on the State of Young People's Health in the European Union* (2000).)

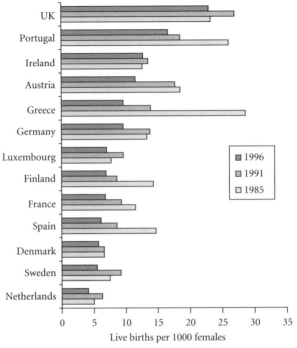

Fig. 1.24 Fertility rates for 15–19 year-olds during 1999. (Source: *EC Report on the State of Young People's Health in the European Union* (2000).)

Clearly the truth lies somewhere between these two extremes. It is now well recognized that health services cannot solve the health problems of the population on their own, and that in some areas social and environmental action are of prime importance. Nonetheless, health services do have a vital role to play in maintaining and improving the public's—and not least children's—health. Inequalities in health are exacerbated by inequalities in access to health care, through an unfair geographical distribution of services (the so-called 'inverse care law') and barriers to access such as lack of interpreters or public transport or limited clinic times.

It is important to be sure that health services—both locally and nationally—promote rather than hinder equity, and that they are effective in meeting the needs of the population. Public health techniques such as health needs assessment and evaluation of services, and the rise in evidence-based medicine, can help to ensure that the country gets best value from the NHS and that it contributes positively to promoting health and reducing health inequalities.

Recent developments in the NHS point the service in this direction. Historically in the UK there has been an excellent primary care service for children, through the provision of home visiting programmes for the preschool child and school health services for the school child. Links to the GP and primary care team ensure that interdisciplinary working is facilitated. However, longstanding divisions between the management of preventive and curative services have meant that there is a lack of integration and often inadequate staffing in community child health (as well as limited evidence of effectiveness).

The current trend is to integrate care between various sectors and to ensure that social and health care are commissioned together. Rhetoric does not always match reality in this field, however, and the role of health professionals as advocates to ensure that services meet the needs of children is vitally important.

Current trends in NHS services for children include:

◆ 'Joined up thinking' in central government, crossing ministerial and departmental boundaries

◆ Greater focus on community and ambulatory care

◆ Primary care led commissioning

◆ Joint commissioning of children's services with local authorities

◆ Local interventions working with communities with the aim of increasing social capital (e.g. 'Sure Start')

◆ Emphasis on team work, with no assumption of medical leadership

◆ Development of nurse autonomy (e.g. nurse practitioners)

◆ Greater partnership with parents and consumer participation in planning

◆ More consultation with children and young people

Clustering of problems

This section has reviewed a range of key factors which impact on children's health. Although each exerts independent effects, it is also the case that many of the factors which adversely affect children's health tend to cluster. Thus children with one problem are often at greater risk of experiencing others, and individual adverse factors may potentiate the effects of others. This phenomenon has been called 'social patterning'. We have seen how adverse social circumstances collectively contribute to a higher risk of teenage pregnancy, which in itself has a negative impact on health for both mother and child, and how children from ethnic minority groups often suffer the effects of poverty as well as intolerance and bullying, while struggling with a new language and culture and difficulties in accessing health and other services. They may also be at greater risk of certain congenital conditions, and possibly of infectious diseases such as HIV and TB which may be prevalent in their country of origin. Similarly, vulnerable children looked after by the local authority are at greater risk of teenage pregnancy, tend to have lower educational achievement, and have often experienced abusive or neglectful family relationships.

Clearly this tendency for clustering of problems compounds the impact on children's health and well-being and exaggerates the health inequalities which result. It is important for child public health practitioners to address individual determinants of health, but they also need to be aware of this tendency for adverse factors to cluster and interact, complicating the picture and requiring a more sophisticated approach to tackling child public health problems.

Table 1.6 Environmental influences on child health

Age	Environmental influences	Outcome
Infant	Parenting sensitivity and attunement to infant needs, nutrition, breast-feeding, housing	Emotional and social development, development of motor skills, speech and language, infections, physical growth, healthly teeth
Preschool child	Parenting style, television exposure, marketing of unhealthy foods, safety of play area, learning environment	Behaviour problems, mental health, language development, accidental injury, cognitive skills, growth, anaemia, abuse, peer group relationships, readiness for school
School-age child	School ethos, parenting style, road safety awareness, television, marketing, sports facilities	Violence, bullying, academic progression, accidental injury, citizenship, physical fitness, depression, behaviour problems, relationship problems
Adolescent	Advertising and media, parental relationships, school ethos, sports facilities, parenting style	Tobacco and substance abuse, relationship problems, sexually transmitted disease, pregnancy, violence, delinquency, criminality

The biopsychosocial environmental framework

Referring to the Mandala diagram earlier in the chapter, the biopsychosocio-environmental framework it describes is helpful in considering the relationship of health and disease to socio-economic and environmental factors. For example, a child with poor growth and development may be found to have the 'diseases' of iron deficiency anaemia and rickets, with impairments in the production of healthy red blood cells and bone disease secondary to calcium and vitamin D deficiency. The cause is often nutritional deficiency associated with delayed weaning and lack of sunlight, which might be related to destitute living circumstances and to poor nutritional knowledge and practice among parents, which are themselves closely related to unemployment and poverty. The level at which disease or pathology is located depends on your viewpoint. Intervention, including prevention, often requires a multi-level approach of the kind described for a range of child public health problems in Chapter 7.

Impact on different age groups through childhood and adolescence

In the previous section we have examined the factors in society which affect children's health. The impact of these factors varies according to the age of the child, and the relationships are illustrated in Table 1.6.

Conclusions

In this chapter we have examined the changes which are taking place in society and how they affect children's health and development in the UK. There is no doubt that many of these changes are beneficial to children and that children's health and well-being are better and more widely protected than was the case a hundred years ago. Educational standards, social support, health care, and knowledge about child development have all improved and child abuse is much less widely tolerated. However, many 'advances' have been harmful to children. Inequalities in wealth and health are a scar on our society and the extent of emotional and behavioural problems indicates that all is not yet right with family relationships. Health professionals need to be aware of these problems, and can help by working with others in society to monitor the effects on children's health and by speaking out strongly to bring them to the attention of policy makers and the government. It is in this area that the emerging discipline of child public health will prove its mettle.

Further reading

Barker, M. and Power, C. (1993). Disability in young adults: the role of injuries. *J Epidemiol Community Health* 47(5):349–54.

Barnes, G. (1984). Adolescent alcohol abuse and other problem behaviors: their relationship and common parental influences. *Journal of Youth and Adolescence* 13:329–84.

Baumrind D. (1967). Child care practices anteceding three patterns of preschool behaviour. *Genetic Psychology Monographs* 75(1):43–88.

Baumrind, D. (1991). Parenting styles and adolescent development. In *The encyclopaedia on adolescence* (R. Learner, A.C. Peteresen, J. Brooks-Gunn, eds.), pp. 746–58. Garland, New York.

British Medical Association (1999). (i) Childhood injury and abuse. (ii) Emotional and behavioural problems. (iii) Inequalities in child health. (iv) Nutrition. In *Growing up in Britain: ensuring a healthy future for our children. A study of 0–5 year olds.* British Medical Association, London.

Chinn, S. and Rona, R.J. (2001). Prevalence and trends in overweight and obesity in three cross sectional studies of British children, 1974–94. *BMJ*; **322**:24–6.

Cohen, D., Richardson, J., and LaBree, L. (1994). Parenting behaviors and the onset of smoking and alcohol use: a longitudinal study. *Pediatrics*; **94**:368–75.

Committee on Integrating the Science of Early Childhood Development (2000). Nurturing relationships. In *From neurons to neighborhoods: the science of early childhood development.* National Academy Press, Washington DC.

Egeland, B., Carlson, E., and Sroufe, L.A. (1993). Resilience as a process. In *Development and psychopathology.* Cambridge University Press, Cambridge.

Harold, G., Pryor, J., and Reynolds, J. (2001). *Not in front of the children.* One plus One Marriage Partnership, The Wells, 7–15 Roseberry Avenue, London EC1R 4SP.

Hart, J.T. (1971). The inverse care law. *Lancet* 1(7696):405–12.

Henricson, C. and Grey, A. (2001). *Understanding discipline: an overview of child discipline practices and their implications for family support.* National Family and Parenting Institute, London.

Innocenti (2000). *A league table of child poverty in rich nations.* Innocenti Research Centre, Florence.

Jacobi A. (1912). The best means of combating infant mortality. *Journal of the American Medical Association* **58**(2):1735–44.

Kohler, L. (1998). Child Public Health: a new basis for child health workers. *Eur J Public Health* **8**:253–5.

Leach, P. (1994). *Children first.* Michael Joseph, London.

Lynch, J.W., Davey Smith, G., Kaplan, G.A., and House, J.S. (2000). Income inequality and mortality: importance to health of individual income, psychosocial environment, or material conditions. *BMJ*; **320**:1200–04.

Paterson, G.R., DeBaryshe, B.D., and Ramsey, E. (1989). A developmental perspective on antisocial behavior. *American Psychologist* **44**(2):329–35.

Platt, M.J. (1998). Child health statistics review. *Archives of Disease in Childhood*; **79**:523–7.

Robinson, T. (1999). Reducing children's TV viewing to prevent obesity. *JAMA*; **282**:1561–7.

Robinson, T.M., Wilde, M.L., Navracruz, L.C., Haydel, K.F., and Varady, A. (2001). Effects of reducing children's television and video game use on aggressive behavior: a randomised controlled trial. *Archives of Pediatric and Adolescent Medicine*; **155**:17–23.

Schore, A.N. (1994). *Affect regulation and the origin of self. The neurobiology of emotional development.* Erlbaum, Hillsdale NJ.

Sharples, P.M., Storey, A., Aynsley–Green, A., and Eyre, J.A. (1990). Causes of fatal childhood accidents involving head injury in northern region. *BMJ*; **301**:1193–7.

Spencer, N.J. (2000). *Poverty and child health.* Radcliffe Press, Oxford.

Sroufe, A. (1996). *Emotional development.* Cambridge University Press, New York.

SUSTAIN (2002). *TV dinners.* SUSTAIN (Campaign for sustainable food and agriculture), London.

Townsend, P. (1999). A structural plan needed to reduce inequalities in health. In *Inequalities in health—the evidence presented to the Independent Enquiry into Inequalities in Health, chaired by Sir Donald Acheson* (ed. Brown, D., Shaw, M., Dorling, D., and Davey Smith, G.). The Policy Press, University of Bristol.

Valman, B. (2000). *The Royal College of Paediatrics and Child Health at the Millennium.* RCPCH.

Weare, K. (2000). *Promoting mental emotional and social health: a whole school approach.* Routledge, London.

Webb, E., Shankleman, J., Evans, M.R., and Brooks, B. (2001). The health of children in refuges for women victims of domestic violence: cross sectional descriptive survey. *BMJ*; **323**:210–13.

Wilkinson, R.G. (1992). Income distribution and life expectancy. *BMJ*; **304**:165–8.

Woodroffe, C., Glickman, M., Barker, M., and Power, C. (1993). *Children teenagers and health: the key data.* Open University Press, Buckingham.

Chapter 2

Child health—the global context

Why is international child health important?

> We must move children to the centre of the world's agenda. We must rewrite strategies to reduce poverty so that investments in children are given priority.
>
> Nelson Mandela

It is hardly possible for anyone in the developed world, lay or professional, to be unaware of the many threats to the health and well-being of children in the developing world. Facts and photographs, crises and appeals populate our newspapers, television screens, and professional journals—especially since the recent growth in global terrorism. Many of us now travel to parts of the world we have previously only read about, and are seeing very different societies at first hand for the first time. Nevertheless, despite our familiarity with images of life in the developing world, there is a risk that we are all too busy with our own everyday lives to acknowledge our part in the global scheme.

It is salutary to remember that roughly 85% of the world's 1.5 billion children live in developing countries, and that the accident of their country of birth marks them out from the beginning for a very different experience of life and health. A comparison of child health indicators between the top five and bottom five countries in the world, as in Table 2.1, provides a stark illustration of the contrast between them. A child born in Sierra Leone has an almost one in three chance of dying before reaching his or her fifth birthday—almost eighty times higher than for a child born in Sweden, Norway, or Japan. Fewer than 20% of the population in Sierra Leone, Niger, Afghanistan, or Mali have adequate sanitation, and barely one in two children in these countries receives basic immunizations.

The key health problems facing children in different parts of the globe differ significantly. Most child deaths worldwide are due to preventable causes such as perinatal conditions, respiratory infections, and diarrhoeal diseases. Many of these are related to poverty and malnutrition, which are both widespread and increasing— and both of which are significantly affected by the behaviour of more developed countries. Immunization has been a success story, but huge numbers of children still die from vaccine-preventable diseases. Obviously some conditions—such as mental illness, disability, and teenage pregnancy—are common to both the developed and developing world, but their prevalence, their impact on the child and family, and the services available to deal with them differ between industrialized countries and those with a subsistence economy. Similarly, many determinants of health—such as housing

Table 2.1 Comparison of child health indicators in different countries (top five and bottom five under fives mortality)

Country	Under 5s mortality (per 1000 births)	Immunization uptake % (DPT/polio)	Exclusive breast-feeding 0–3 months	% of population with adequate sanitation	Rank
Sierra Leone	316	56	–	11	1
Angola	292	36	12	40	2
Niger	280	22	1	19	3
Afghanistan	257	35	25	10	4
Mali	237	52	13	6	5
France	5	97	–	–	175
Singapore	5	96	–	–	175
Japan	4	99	–	85	189
Norway	4	92	–	–	189
Sweden	4	99	–	–	189

(– means data unavailable) Source: UNICEF (2000) *State of the World's Children*

conditions and family structure—are relevant to all children worldwide, but their nature, severity, and relative impact on health varies. Table 2.2 highlights some of the contrasts.

So why should we, as individuals concerned with child public health, know more about children growing up in less privileged countries? Do we have responsibilities towards them, and can we do anything to improve their health and well-being? Does the situation in far-flung parts of the globe have an impact on our own practice? Could a better understanding of the background to migration and asylum seeking, for example, help us to plan and provide health services at home?

This chapter aims to answer these and other questions, offering an international perspective on children in society and their health, exploring the complex links between different parts of the globe and arguing that there is significant inter-dependence between them. It discusses the key health problems of children who live in developing countries where poverty and lack of resources are key mediators, as well as those whose lives have been disrupted by war and infrastructure breakdown, and examines some of the solutions which have been developed through research or innovations in practice—some of which could benefit child public health practice in the developed world too.

This is an enormous subject which is inevitably covered here in summary only, but we hope this chapter offers some insight into what we consider to be a vitally

Table 2.2 Comparison of some important determinants of health and key health problems in children in the developed and developing world

	Developed world	Developing world
Important determinants of health	Inappropriate nutrition e.g. overconsumption of saturated fats and sugar Lack of exercise Risk behaviour e.g. substance misuse Relative poverty/income inequality Family structure and relationships Social attitudes and stigma Time spent watching TV/playing video games	Malnutrition Absolute poverty Lack of sanitation Availability of education War and conflict Famine, drought, and flooding Availability of health care, especially antenatal, perinatal, and preventive services Family planning and family size Child labour Migration
Key health problems	Acute illnesses (usually not fatal) Obesity Emotional and behavioural problems Disability (a significant proportion due to increasing survival of preterm infants) Chronic illnesses	Respiratory infections Diarrhoeal diseases Vaccine-preventable infectious diseases and other acute illnesses (more often fatal) HIV, TB, and Hepatitis B Disability (more often caused by accidents or by war and conflict)

important area of child public health and that it will be of interest and relevance to readers from all backgrounds.

The global burden of childhood disease

Child health problems in developing countries today are not dissimilar to those seen in Europe in the eighteenth and nineteenth century, both in terms of the extent and severity of ill health and of the range of conditions encountered. The diseases of poverty, and common infectious diseases which have largely been conquered in the developed north, are more significant than tropical diseases. The new 'plagues' of the twentieth and twenty-first centuries, especially HIV, mental illness, and injury have added dramatically to the burden of disease, whilst the mitigating effect of socioeconomic, environmental, and technological progress has had little impact in many countries.

Children in developing countries today face similar health problems to European children in previous centuries—diseases of poverty and common infectious diseases—but to these are added the new 'plagues' of HIV, mental illness, and injury.

In Europe and the USA, infant mortality is now below 10 per 1000 births, but in many developing countries it remains above 100 per 1000 births, and in some cases is as high as 300. The most common causes of infant death in such countries are septicaemia, tetanus of the newborn, birth injury from unskilled midwifery, low birth weight, and congenital malformations.

Almost 11 million children under five died last year in developing countries, most from preventable causes. In 1998, the major causes of death in this group were perinatal conditions (20%), respiratory infections (18%), diarrhoeal diseases (17%), vaccine-preventable infectious diseases (15%—including measles, which alone accounted for 5% of deaths), and malaria (7%). Malnutrition is implicated in more than half of children's deaths worldwide. The impact of malnutrition is discussed further below, in the section on determinants of health.

Most child deaths worldwide are due to preventable causes such as perinatal conditions, respiratory infections, and diarrhoeal diseases, many of them related to poverty and malnutrition. Immunization has been a success story, but huge numbers of children still die from vaccine-preventable diseases.

Diseases related to or exacerbated by poverty

The extent and impact of poverty is discussed in detail in the next section, on determinants of health. Some of the diseases associated with poverty are illustrated in the box below:

- Malnutrition—which has direct and indirect effects on health (e.g. starvation, vitamin deficiency, and greater susceptibility to disease)
- Diarrhoeal disease
- Acute respiratory infections (measles, pertussis, pneumonia)
- Tuberculosis
- HIV infection
- Skin and eye infections

Common infectious diseases

Many common infectious diseases—most of them now rare causes of death or serious illness in developed countries—remain major killers in poor countries. Measles is a particularly significant example, accounting for 5% of deaths in children under five in developing countries. Measles is more severe in malnourished children, especially those with vitamin A deficiency, and the risk of serious complications is much higher. Whereas the death rate from measles in developed countries is only 2–3 per 1000 cases, in developing countries it is at least 30–50 per 1000 cases, and may be as high as 100–300 per 1000 cases in some areas. This variation is probably due to a greater intensity of infecting dose owing to overcrowding, rather than a different virus.

The worldwide prevalence of tuberculosis includes 2 billion people infected and 16 million active cases. The vast majority live in high prevalence areas (with more than 40 cases per 100,000 population) such as Africa, South and South East Asia, and South America, and a substantial proportion of them are children. The risk of active disease following infection is high in children under three, those with poor nutritional status and living conditions, and specifically in HIV-positive individuals, for whom the risk is increased ten-fold. Effective treatment requires the use of at least three drugs for several months, which may be difficult to achieve.

Hepatitis B is also a significant problem in many countries, with over 2 billion people infected worldwide and over a million deaths per year. In countries with high prevalence (over 8% of the population) such as Africa, many children are affected, usually by transmission from mother to baby at birth. Children are more likely to become chronic carriers of the virus and to suffer long-term complications such as cirrhosis or cancer of the liver.

Acute respiratory infections, meningitis, and other potentially treatable or preventable diseases are also more common (and often more serious) in developing countries. Lack of availability of what we might consider basic medicines—such as antibiotics—compromise the outcome for children already made more vulnerable to serious disease by poor nutrition and general health.

Immunization was the success story of the twentieth century: smallpox has been eradicated worldwide, and many countries have reduced the burden of measles, polio, and pertussis by effective immunization programmes. Polio could be eradicated by 2005: in 2001 there were 483 reported cases of polio worldwide, down from 350,000 in 1988. However, the potential benefits of immunization have not been fully realised. Fewer than half of children in certain parts of Africa currently receive measles vaccine, for example. Problems with vaccine delivery and uptake are discussed further in the section on determinants of health.

> 2–3 children die per 1000 cases of measles in developed countries, compared to up to 300 per 1000 cases in some developing countries. TB and Hepatitis B also remain common and potentially serious causes of ill health worldwide.

AIDS and HIV infection

The current global AIDS epidemic is a tragedy for children as well as for their families. 36.1 million people were estimated to be living with AIDS at the end of 2000, and 95% of them live in the developing world. The overall worldwide distribution is shown in Figure 2.1.

At the end of 1999, 1.3 million children worldwide were living with HIV and 3.8 million children had died since the beginning of the epidemic. 250,000 children

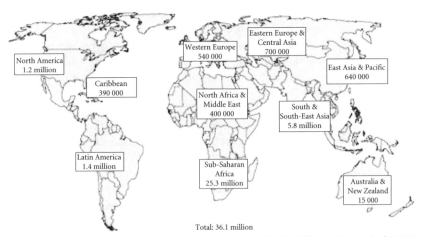

Fig. 2.1 Adults and children estimated to be living with AIDS/HIV at the end of 2000. (Source: Grant, A. and De Cock, K. *BMJ* (2001) **322**:1475–8, with permission from the BMJ Publishing Group.)

acquire the HIV virus every month. Roughly 10% of all new infections are in children under 15, and 50% are in young people aged 15–24. Almost all children with HIV under 15 years old acquired the infection through vertical transmission from their mothers, at birth or immediately after. Although studies have shown that vertical transmission can be virtually eliminated with antiretroviral therapy, the expense and lack of availability of these drugs in many countries means that enormous numbers of HIV-positive mothers and their babies fail to benefit from them. Major questions and obstacles remain to be addressed before HIV in children can be successfully prevented and treated.

As well as the direct effects of infection in children, the impact of losing relatives to AIDS is also devastating, with many children being left in charge of families and younger siblings at a young age.

> 1.3 million children were living with HIV, and 3.8 million children had died from the disease, at the end of the twentieth century. Most caught it through vertical transmission from their mothers, which can be prevented with antiretroviral therapy.

Injuries

If one examines the global burden of disease in terms of disability adjusted life years (DALYs), then injuries come second only to infectious disease, and constitute, for example, seven times the burden of disease of nutritional deficiency.

More than 85% of all deaths and 90% of disability adjusted life years lost from road traffic injuries occur in developing countries. In 1998, among children aged 0–4 and 5–14 years, the number of fatalities per 100,000 population in low-income

Table 2.3 Burden of disease for various conditions worldwide

Disease category	Burden of disease in 2000 (1000 DALYs)
Infectious and parasitic disease	131,327
Injuries	58,352
Perinatal conditions	18,700
Neuropsychiatric conditions	15,788
Nutritional deficiency	8389
Malignant conditions	8114
Congenital anomalies	5224

Adapted from Murray, C.J.L. and Lopez, A.D. (1996). *Global burden of disease: a comprehensive assessment of mortality and disability from diseases, injuries, and risk factors in 1990 and projected to 2020.* Harvard School of Public Health, Boston, MA; World Health Organization, World Bank.

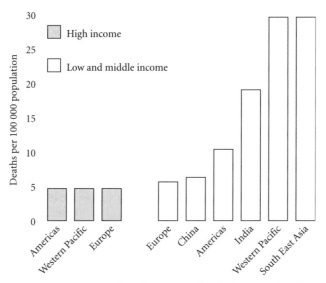

Fig. 2.2 Fatality rates due to road traffic injuries in children aged 0–4 years, 1998. (Source: World Health Organization, *BMJ* (2002) **324**:1140, with permission from the BMJ Publishing Group.)

countries was about six times greater than in high-income countries—including a fourfold greater proportion of children killed as pedestrians.

The main reasons for these inequalities are the growth of numbers of motor vehicles, higher numbers of deaths and injuries per crash, poor enforcement of traffic safety regulations, inadequacy of public health service infrastructure, and poor access to public health care.

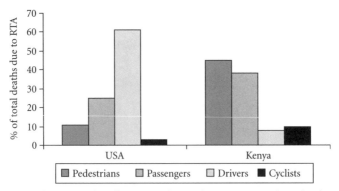

Fig. 2.3 Deaths due to road traffic injuries by road user category in a developed and a developing country. (Source: World Health Organization, *BMJ* (2002) **324**:1140, with permission from the BMJ Publishing Group.)

Reproductive health

In older children, teenage pregnancy remains a particularly worrying issue. Nearly 15 million girls aged 15–19 years give birth each year, accounting for more than 10% of all babies born worldwide.

In many developing countries, more than one-third of women continue to give birth in their teens. This has a major impact on health, with the risk of death from pregnancy-related causes being four times higher in this age group than for women over the age of 20 years.

Tropical diseases

As well as the more familiar infectious diseases discussed above, children in many parts of the world are at risk of tropical diseases which can cause death, disability, or severe illness. Some of the more important are listed in the box below:

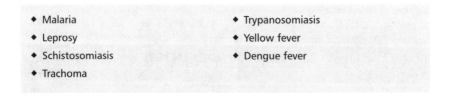

- Malaria
- Leprosy
- Schistosomiasis
- Trachoma
- Trypanosomiasis
- Yellow fever
- Dengue fever

Malaria is a major cause of illness and death in certain areas where the more severe falciparum malaria remains endemic, including Brazil, South East Asia, and sub-Saharan Africa (where 90% of deaths occur). It can lead to serious complications and, if untreated, the mortality rate in children may reach 40%. The other types of malaria are rarely fatal but can lead to protracted, even lifelong infection, with intermittent relapses.

Leprosy, too, is still a significant problem, affecting over a million people worldwide, including upwards of 5 per 1000 population in some tropical and subtropical countries. Although uncommon in children under three (partly because of its long incubation period), it is seen in older children, and cases do occur even in infancy, probably due to transplacental transmission. Its major impact is in terms of the disfigurement and disability resulting from chronic infection. As for tuberculosis, treatment is possible but needs to be long-term—at least 12 months of multidrug therapy.

For parasitic infections such as schistosomiasis (bilharzia), the most serious consequences are generally those of chronic infection, which include liver fibrosis, intractable urinary obstruction, and infertility. Trachoma infection in childhood frequently leads to blindness in later life; it is widespread in many parts of the world, including northern and sub-Saharan Africa, parts of Asia, and South America. Trypanosomiasis (sleeping sickness) is confined to tropical Africa, where the tsetse fly is found, and is always fatal without treatment: one form kills within weeks, whereas the other may last for years before finally leading to death.

Yellow fever and Dengue fever—both transmitted by mosquitoes—cause acute illness, with a fatality rate which is generally below 5%, although the more severe form of Dengue is more common in children. They have recently been joined by several newer types of viral haemorrhagic fever including Lassa and Ebola.

Disability

The burden of untreated disability in children in developing countries is significant. The causes include the exotic (leprosy and other tropical diseases) and the more familiar (meningitis and other infections, traffic accidents, war, landmines, congenital abnormalities, and birth injuries); many of them are preventable or treatable. The manifestations may be physical (including problems with vision and hearing as well as locomotor impairments) or psychological. Few data are available on mental health problems but these are manifest in association with war, separation and displacement, child exploitation, and child labour. It is likely that they represent a very significant burden which will be recognized as awareness grows.

> The burden of untreated disability in children in developing countries is significant. Lack of surgical facilities, therapists, and adaptive aids and devices means many of those affected do not reach their potential. The impact of their lost labour may be very significant for themselves and their families.

There is a great need for increased emphasis on disability in the training of health workers and the operation of the services.

Determinants of health in children in low-income countries

Environmental and socioeconomic factors are the most significant determinants of disease, and poverty is increasing in many countries, particularly in Africa. This

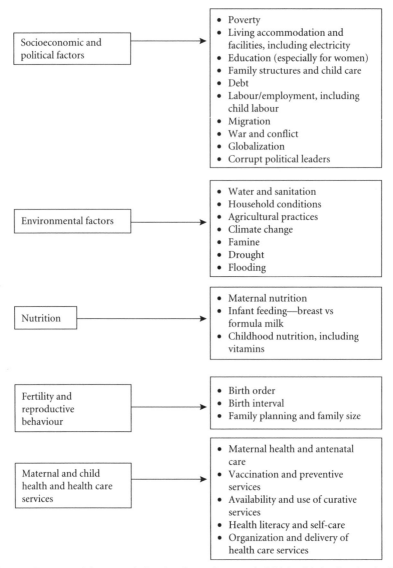

Fig. 2.4 Conceptual framework for the determinants of child health in the developing world. (Source: Adapted from Dabis, F., Orne-Gliemann, J., Perez, F. *et al*. *BMJ* (2002) **324**:1444–7, with permission from the BMJ Publishing Group.)

increase is related to the trade and aid policies of industrialized countries. Health care programmes are often based on models adopted from industrialized countries which may not be appropriate. Figure 2.4 represents the determinants of health in developing countries.

Key determinants of health in children in developing countries are environmental and socioeconomic factors—many of them (including poverty, globalization, and climate change) affected by the behaviour of industrialized countries.

Some of these factors are explored in greater detail below.

Poverty

Poverty is the greatest problem facing children who live in developing countries. The box below illustrates the extent of global poverty, which is severe and worsening, although some countries are succeeding in mitigating its effects. The extent of change is shown by the fact that two centuries ago, income per head in Britain, the world's richest country at that time, was three times higher than that of Africa, then the planet's poorest region. Today, the world's richest country, Switzerland, enjoys per capita income nearly 80 times higher than the world's poorest region, south Asia (*The Guardian*, 22nd August 2002)

1.3 billion people live on less than $1 a day

Of the 4.4 billion people living in developing countries:

    — three fifths lack access to sanitation

    — one third lack clean water

    — one fifth have no health care

    — one fifth do not have enough dietary energy and protein

The world's 225 richest people have a combined wealth equivalent to the annual income of the poorest 2.5 billion (nearly half the world's population)

Source: *BMJ* (1997) 314:529

As in developed countries, poverty affects health through a wide variety of mechanisms and diseases, although its effects are more stark in countries where absolute poverty is severe.

Lack of access to the basic necessities of life increases susceptibility to ill health (e.g. via malnutrition) and exposure to disease (e.g. via contaminated water supplies), and reduces the capacity to respond to it (including ability to access health care).

In some ways it is better to be poor in a country with a subsistence economy where the majority live in the same situation, than in a country where the majority are well off. However, there are now increasing inequalities within developing countries as well as between rich and poor countries—a relatively new socioeconomic feature which has significantly worsened the situation for the poor. Some of the factors behind this are shown in the box below.

Factors increasing inequalities within developing countries

- Home government policies such as rapid industrialization, military spending, corruption
- Urbanization, which increases poverty by moving families from subsistence to the cash economy and increases environmental degradation
- Government debt and structural adjustment policies imposed by the World Bank, reducing the extent of public services and sometimes introducing user charges for health services which affect the poor more than the rich
- Marketing of unhealthy products such as infant formula milk by multinational corporations, which the poor cannot afford but feel entrained to purchase
- Rapid population growth and demographic entrapment (when a community's requirements exceed the capacity of the land to support them, as well as exceed the capacity to migrate to other regions and their economic capacity to buy food and other essentials)

Reference: Carnall, D. (1999)

Poor families, and especially mothers and children, have suffered most in the transition from a labour intensive, agricultural economy to a capital intensive, urban economy. Education and health services have not kept up with population growth, and infrastructure development has been inadequate to provide for basic needs. Consequently, health has suffered.

Education

Education is a vital determinant of health in developing countries. As well as the direct benefits of education (for example, in terms of future earning power), primary education, especially for women, leads to lower infant mortality rates and longer life expectancy. As little as one or two years of schooling for girls can significantly reduce child mortality when these girls reach child-bearing age: a 10% increase in female literacy reduces child mortality by 10% (whereas increases in male literacy have little impact). Yet worldwide, 125 million children are not attending school, two thirds of them girls; half of Africa's children either do not enter primary school or drop out before finishing (*The Guardian*, 22nd August 2002).

Universal primary education is one of the UN's eight anti-poverty goals, and the cost of achieving it is $7–8 billion a year—the equivalent of four days of military spending around the world.

Family structures and child care

For a family living on the land in a country such as Uganda or India, the quality of life in past generations may have been reasonable. The extended family ensured that child care was always available, locally grown food was adequate, and a strong local culture of music, dance, and history gave children a sense of their roots. Life was hard but the family provided a close and loving environment. Social capital (see Chapter 4) was high and this had beneficial effects on health. However, migration into cities and the breakdown of family structures (exacerbated in many countries by the impact of HIV) have undermined the traditional strengths of these communities.

Debt

Debts incurred by many developing countries (particularly in Africa) following the boom in oil prices in the 1970s led to a situation where many countries were paying more in interest charges to the developed world than they received in aid and revenue. The World Bank and International Monetary Fund will provide loans but their condition is a structural adjustment policy (see box below) which requires the country to cut back on public spending on health and education, with severely adverse effects on the poor. Attempts are now being made to alleviate the global debt situation but many very poor countries still face pressure to limit public spending.

World debt and structural adjustment

- At the end of 1998 developing countries owed $2,465.1 billion to the developed world
- The total debt of sub-Saharan countries is equal to 68% of their GDP
- A condition for loans by the IMF or World Bank is the imposition of structural adjustment policies

Structural adjustment policies include:

- Trade liberalization
- Removal of food subsidies for the poor
- Reduction of public spending on welfare and on education and health services
- The introduction of user charges for health and education

Source: BMA (2000)

Child labour

Worldwide, about 250 million children are engaged in work, often over long hours and in hazardous circumstances. Their health suffers from this both directly and indirectly: via loss of schooling, inappropiate physical stresses, inadequate nutrition, and the physical and psychological effects of 'lost childhood' (taking on excessive responsibilities and forgoing opportunities for play and exercise). Many labouring children are employed by corporations based in rich countries, which have a responsibility for curtailing the practice whilst helping to develop educational alternatives. It is important to understand that a poor family's income may depend on the working child, so banning work without introducing economic alternatives will be opposed by local people. Solutions should be comprehensive and should entail the elimination of hazardous child labour and the provision of free education, together with wider legal protection for children.

Many of the 20 million working children worldwide are employed by multinational corporations. Curtailing child labour—especially child prostitution—is an essential part of promoting children's rights.

Child prostitution is a particularly damaging practice which is being increasingly recognized in many parts of the world. It has serious adverse effects on both mental and physical health, and on life opportunities. The risk of HIV and other sexually transmitted diseases, as well as of teenage pregnancy, are particular hazards for such children.

Children's rights are persistently abused in many countries of the world. The relationship between human rights and health is very close—health workers need to understand and make use of the legal protection provided by the UN Convention on the Rights of the Child (see later in 'Solutions' section).

War and conflict

In recent years wars have occurred in most regions of the world—the majority in developing countries, although recently parts of Europe (especially the former Soviet Union and former Yugoslavia) have been substantially affected. War affects children as victims, direct and indirect, and as combatants (child soldiers). Its impact is frequently devastating, and prevention of conflict must rank as a top priority for action to protect children.

In war, children die, are severely disabled, and suffer grave mental health effects as a result of the loss of parents and relatives. Human rights abuses are common, and children may witness (or experience) rape, torture, and murder. Family and community networks are disrupted, and the social and political infrastructure often breaks down, leading to the loss of even basic health care and other services. Any services which remain may be severely overstretched dealing with war casualties, so that preventive services such as immunization are interrupted. Children may be left homeless, orphaned, and having to take care of younger siblings, and the perils may continue beyond the end of the conflict if landmines remain in the area. The box below summarizes recent data on the effects of war on children.

Effects of war and conflict on children worldwide

- Up to 2 million children have been killed in war in the last 10 years
- 4 million children have been permanently disabled
- 1 million children have been orphaned
- 12 million children have been displaced
- 0.5 million children have died following sanctions in Iraq (WHO data)

Source: *Arch. Dis. Children* (1998) **78**:72–7

Useful websites: Medact.org; IPPNW.org; www.icbl.org; www.mag.org.uk

Migration and refugees

A further consequence of war and conflict, and also of economic pressure, is migration. In 1999 alone, 31 million refugees sought refuge from conflict zones around the world. The vast majority of those fleeing their homeland seek refuge in neighbouring countries as poor as their own, which can have a serious impact on already overstretched economies and services. In industrialized countries, which (contrary to the prevalent publicity) receive a small proportion of all refugees and asylum seekers, these individuals are often seen as scroungers, labelled as 'bogus' asylum seekers, and are subject to racism and harassment as well as to sometimes oppressive government policies. Barriers to entry for asylum seekers are increasing across western Europe, and there is a real risk that the protection and rights offered by the UN Convention on Refugees will be compromised in some countries. Some of the factors affecting the health of refugees and asylum seekers are shown in the box below:

Factors affecting the health of refugees and asylum seekers

- Previous life experiences e.g. war, torture, bereavement, perilous flight
- Loss of family networks and community
- Disrupted health care in home country
- For some, increased risk of infectious diseases (including TB and HIV)
- Impact of poverty and social exclusion in host country
- Impact of racism and discrimination in host country
- Effect of being part of ethnic minority in host country
- Poor access to health care services in host country due to lack of understanding of needs, availability, and entitlements (among staff as well as users), and to language and cultural barriers

The combined health impact of these factors is considerable. Support from health and other services is essential for this vulnerable group in the population. In the UK, asylum seekers and refugees are entitled to receive NHS services in the same way as other residents, and local commissioners have a responsibility to ensure that they have equitable access to appropriate services, including the provision of interpreters, information about NHS services (which may differ substantially from those in their country of origin), and special services (where necessary to cater for particular needs such as mental health problems). Training for health care staff is also essential, and published resources are available to support this.

Children, especially unaccompanied children, are a particularly vulnerable subgroup with high rates of mental health problems as a result of their experiences. The UK has excluded asylum seeking children from its ratification of the UN Convention on the Rights of the Child, compromising their rights compared to indigenous children. Although they are offered some protection by the Children Act and other legislation, this ceases when they reach eighteen, so their ability to build a new life in this country may be undermined.

Globalization

This term has been coined to describe the universalization of trade, culture, and communication that has developed across the globe in recent years. It has its origins in the worldwide market in commodities, led by multinational corporations, and the explosion of international communication as a result of the spread of TV and the development of the internet. The key elements of globalization, and the impact some aspects of globalization have on children, are illustrated in the boxes below.

Key elements of globalization

- The growth of transnational corporations such as Nike, Nestle, and Esso, many of which are larger in terms of economic productivity than some single countries and have huge marketing budgets
- The domination of the media and communications industry by a few companies such as CNN and News International, which has led to the international dissemination of media icons such as sports and music celebrities and the emphasis on a mainly Western lifestyle in images presented across the world, and increased awareness of poverty and disadvantage among those in developing countries
- The internet, which has revolutionized communication and access to information
- The growth of civil society with local community-based movements of people united by a common interest (e.g. the Narmada Movement which has opposed the damming of the Narmada River in North India)

Multinational corporations: good or bad for children?

Beneficial effects	Adverse effects
Reduction in price of consumer goods in industrialized countries	Child labour
	Marketing of unhealthy products
Wide availability and choice of quality products	Unethical marketing (e.g. infant formula milk)
	Lack of regulation by legislation
	Pressure to buy (fashion)

The internet: good or bad for children?

Beneficial effects	Adverse effects
Education	As TV (see Chapter 5)
Encourages self-learning	Easy access to pornography
Promotes international networking	Inappropriate cultural images

It will be a challenge for civil society to develop ways of controlling multinational corporations and ensuring that children are protected from the adverse effects of the internet, in particular pornography and other sexual imagery.

Environmental factors

Environmental factors such as sudden changes in climate, resulting in flooding and breaches in sanitation maintenance, can have devastating effects on the population and on the socioeconomic stability of a country. Crop production may be wiped out within a few days and leave a country dependent on outside aid and support. Floods and crop damage lead in turn to malnutrition and outbreaks of infectious diseases such as cholera and typhoid fever.

Malnutrition and vitamin deficiencies

Much of the difference in mortality between the developed and developing world is mediated by malnutrition. Over 50% of the world's malnourished children and low birth weight infants live in south Asia, and one in three of Africa's children are underweight. It is estimated that 226 million children worldwide are stunted by malnutrition which, as we have already seen, has a major impact on their ability to resist and recover from infection.

Nutritional deficiencies in minerals and vitamins are estimated to cost some countries the equivalent of more than 5% of their GNP in lost lives, disability, and productivity.

Table 2.4 Maternal and child malnutrition 1990–8

Area	% infants with low birth weight 1990–7	% children with wasting	% maternal anaemia
Latin America and Carribean	9	3	30
Middle East and North Africa	11	8	50
Sub-Saharan Africa	15	9	50
East Asia and the Pacific	10	n/a	40
South Asia	33	18	75
Developing countries	18	11	56
Industrialized countries	6	<1	18

(Source: Bhutta, Z.A. *BMJ* (2000) **321**:810–12, with permission from the BMJ Publishing Group.)

The specific impact of nutritional deficiencies in minerals and vitamins was the subject of a 1998 UNICEF report. Night-blindness due to vitamin A deficiency affects 10–20% of women worldwide, and vitamin A supplementation can lead to 38% fewer maternal deaths. In children, vitamin A deficiency is a significant cause of blindness and increases mortality rates from other diseases such as measles and diarrhoea.

The 1990 World Summit for Children singled out iron, iodide, and vitamin A deficiencies as the most important and amenable to action. In Georgia, widespread iodide deficiency is estimated to have robbed the country of 500,000 IQ points in the 50,000 babies born in 1996 alone. Zinc deficiency is increasingly recognized, as is vitamin D deficiency, especially in Mongolia and other countries of the Commonwealth of Independent States where the winters are long.

Infant feeding

Except for HIV-positive mothers, for whom it carries a significant risk of passing infection to the baby, breast-feeding is overwhelmingly the best method of infant feeding for all countries across the world. The risks of formula-feeding are increased in developing countries, where access to safe water supplies may be limited and advice on appropriate feed composition may not be available. Moreover, the expense of purchasing formula may be crippling for poor families. Manufacturers seeking to expand their market often exploit perceptions of formula-feeding as more sophisticated and 'Western', and therefore desirable; they may provide free supplies for maternity hospitals, hoping to get babies and mothers established on bottle-feeding before discharge. They also attempt to influence doctors and nurses, through gifts and sponsorship, to prescribe their products, and this marketing is remarkably effective.

> Unless mothers are HIV-positive, breast-feeding is the best method of infant feeding for all countries. The risks of formula-feeding are greater in developing countries.

Fertility and reproductive behaviour

Large family size is a distinctive feature in most low-income countries and has been the focus of much aid and education by industrialized countries. This has often been ineffective because of inappropriate targeting, and there is now much wider understanding of how reproductive decisions are taken. The key factors in reducing family size are increasing income (so that children are not seen as an economic necessity), educating women, and making contraceptive advice available throughout the health service. Countries such as Kerala (a state of Southern India) and Sri Lanka, which have focussed on these factors, have had remarkable success in fertility reduction. Family size and short birth interval are important predictors of nutritional status, but far more of the earth's resources are used by the small families of the industrialized countries rather than the large families of the poor world.

Health care

There are substantial problems with the financing and provision of health care in developing countries. As in the industrialized world, the cost of drugs and hospital care is ever-increasing, while the budgets for health services remain static or shrink. All countries face a conflict over the priorities for health care provision, but this is heightened in low-income countries. The box below illustrates some of the dilemmas faced by developing countries:

Problems in health care in developing countries

- High cost of drugs and investigations
- Pressure on doctors to prescribe expensive drugs—drug companies play a role in promoting costly alternatives to simple, cheap drugs and in limiting the availability of low cost generic medicines
- Pressure from some sections of the population to expand hospital and curative services at the expense of primary and preventive services
- Pressure from doctors seeking higher salaries
- 'Brain drain' of doctors to industrialized countries
- Training of doctors orientates them to curative care rather than to prevention, and to individual consultation rather than teamwork and a population approach
- Relatively low spending on primary care
- Poor management in primary care
- Pressure from the World Bank, IMF, and World Trade Organisation to introduce user charges

As a result of pressure from government officials, doctors, and the general public, a high proportion of health budgets go into the secondary and tertiary sector to the detriment of primary health care, although it is through the latter that the main health benefits for the poor will accrue. This can lead to a situation where basic health care for the majority of the population is poor, but 'high tech' hospitals in the large cities can provide expensive state of the art treatment for a small minority of wealthy citizens. These tensions are present in all countries but are more urgent in poor countries where the health problems are so much more serious. A good example of the way in which primary care service organization can impact on health outcome is in the delivery of vaccination and the utilization of 'low tech' oral rehydration for diarrhoeal diseases.

Immunization

Table 2.5 illustrates immunization uptake and the financing of vaccine by governments in different regions of the world. There is not a clear relationship between the two, suggesting that other issues need to be considered. These include supply and administration including the disrupting effect of war, insufficiently trained primary care staff, or poor cold chain supply (the essential process by which vaccine is kept sufficiently cold to prevent deterioration between manufacture and delivery to patients). One potential problem is that immunization delivery is often organized centrally and may not be well integrated with primary care systems.

Table 2.5 Immunization coverage and vaccine supply

Area	% of routine vaccines financed by government	% fully immunized	
		TB	DPT
Sub-Saharan Africa	51	63	48
Middle East and North Africa	83	89	89
South Asia	95	77	70
East Asia and Pacific	94	92	89
Latin America and Caribbean	97	92	85
CEE/CIS and Baltic States	–	91	93
Industrialized countries	–	–	94
Developing countries	85	81	72
Least developed countries	36	70	54
World	85	82	74

Source: UNICEF (2000) *State of the World's Children*

Pharmaceutical supplies

Pharmaceutical supplies are a major difficulty for developing countries. Much less research is undertaken on the development of new drugs for high prevalence diseases in poor countries than on drugs to alleviate disorders which are common in developed countries. Only 16 out of 1393 new medicines brought to market between 1975 and 1999 were for tropical diseases and TB; it was 13 times more likely that a new drug would be for cancer or a central nervous system disorder than for one of the diseases taking such a toll in poor countries.

Drug supplies may be too expensive for developing countries without their own pharmaceutical industries. The major drug companies resist the use of cheaper generic drugs, which has been a major issue in relation to treatment for HIV and AIDS. There is also a tendency for doctors to prescribe new expensive drugs rather than older cheaper ones, perhaps as a result of the marketing inducements used by pharmaceutical companies. WHO has developed an essential drug list: these drugs should be used in preference to newer and more expensive alternatives.

Several factors affect the availability of pharmaceuticals in poor countries. Drugs are expensive to import, especially if pharmaceutical companies resist the use of cheaper generic alternatives. Fewer new drugs are developed for the conditions which most affect developing countries.

There are also difficult issues to confront in terms of weighing up the benefits and disadvantages of certain interventions. For example, the use of rotavirus vaccine has not been pursued in the US because it carries a risk of complications (intestinal intus-susception) which might outweigh the benefits in that country. But in developing countries, where the morbidity and mortality associated with rotaviral gastroenteritis in children are so much greater, the potential health benefits of the vaccine may substantially exceed the risk of side-effects. However, there are concerns about the ethics and stigma of promoting interventions and drugs rejected by rich countries in poorer ones.

Making the links between north and south

Despite the enormous discrepancies between children's health and well-being in developed and developing countries, and the apparent chasm between the two, there are many interconnections between different parts of the globe and many ways in which practices and behaviour in the northern hemisphere affect child health in the southern hemisphere. Some of these are illustrated in the box below.

Connections between developed and developing countries

- Training overseas doctors in the UK may encourage 'brain drain' (but can increase expertise in developing countries if schemes which encourage doctors to return home, such as short-term placements and studentships, are used)
- Donating expensive medical equipment may encourage inappropriate use of 'high tech' health care
- Buying global products such as clothing may promote child labour
- Buying infant formula company products may promote use of bottle-feeding in poor countries
- Export of landmines can disable children
- Excessive use of fossil fuels leads to global warming and increased child deaths due to flooding and more vector-based disease
- Certain health problems in developing countries can impact on northern countries through imported diseases e.g. malaria, HIV
- Policies of transnational corporations favour populations in industrialized countries and have a negative effect in poor countries
- Arms trade always harms children
- Trade policies which favour the rich and harm the poor

Responsibilities of the north

Many of the economic problems facing children in developing countries are the result of patterns of consumption which exist in the richer developed countries. Consumers in the north may be unaware of the impact their behaviour has on people (especially children) in poorer countries. The box below illustrates some of the priorities in spending in rich countries and how the same spending might have benefited children globally.

Misplaced priorities? Annual expenditure on selected items

Basic education for all would cost	*$6bn*	
Current spending on cosmetics in the US		$8bn
Water and sanitation for all would cost	*$9bn*	
Current spending on ice cream in Europe		$11bn
Reproductive health for all women would cost	*$12bn*	
Current spending on pet foods in Europe		$17bn
Basic health and nutrition for all would cost	*$13bn*	
Current spending on cigarettes in Europe		$50bn
Current world military expenditure		$780bn

Source: Human Development Report 1999

What can the north learn from the south?

Despite the frequent assumption that the 'trade' in expertise tends to be one way, with richer industrialized countries leading the way, there are a number of ways in which developments and concepts originating in poorer countries have had (or could have) a positive impact on practice in the northern hemisphere. Some of these are listed in the box below.

Significant innovations pioneered in the developing world

- Oral rehydration therapy (ORT) use in cases of diarrhoea, which originated in the developing world, has been a success story worldwide and is now used in most countries. It is one of the key interventions which has been exported from the southern hemisphere and is increasingly being used in primary care and hospital practice in the developed world.
- The use of personal child health records, which originated in West Africa, is now well established in many developed countries.
- The refocussing on primary care-led services which has occurred in recent years in the UK owes much to models established in other parts of the world.
- Child to child 'peer teaching' methods were pioneered in developing countries and have much potential in terms of health promotion.
- Community development techniques were first used in developing countries (e.g. the use of community members and resources to support initiatives, and the value of local co-operatives).
- Comparative studies of health and of factors such as diet, health care provision, and lifestyle in different parts of the world, and migration studies examining the effects of changes in diet and liefstyle, have provided useful epidemiological information about common diseases and the impact of certain aspects of health care.
- Cultural values such as respect for elders in the community, the importance of family networks, and respect for natural resources are of great potential benefit to richer countries which have progressed so far along the road to industrialization and materialism that they have lost sight of them.

In addition, greater understanding of child health issues in other parts of the world, and of economic, political, and cultural issues in developing countries, could improve health care practice in developed countries in relation to children from ethnic and religious minorities, especially for new arrivals such as asylum seekers and refugees (see earlier section). Important issues include providing professional interpreters, grasping the fact that individuals from the same country may have been on opposite sides of a conflict, and understanding patterns of morbidity in those recently arrived from abroad. Understanding cultural issues is also important, especially in relation to nutrition, women's health (which impacts on child health), family structures, and child rearing. The devaluing of traditional foods can be detrimental to child health, but ascribing too much to 'traditional' child discipline practices can open the door to sanctioning child abuse.

Some solutions to global child health problems

Despite the gloomy picture painted in this chapter, there is much which can be done to improve global child health. The health problems of the developing world today are in many ways similar to those prevalent in Europe two centuries ago, and the answers are similar: less poverty; better nutrition; better housing; better education; clean water, hygiene, and sewage; better basic (and especially preventive) health care. Each of the determinants of health discussed earlier in the chapter can and should be addressed—and although it is neither right nor possible for every solution to be done 'by' the developed world 'to' the developing world, there is nonetheless much that we can do to help, in particular by reducing practices at home which are currently detrimental to other parts of the world.

Some solutions require action at national or international level; others fall within the capabilities of concerned individuals, both lay and professional. The box below sets out some of the approaches which may be beneficial, and the rest of this section explores a few important areas in greater detail.

International measures to improve global child health

- Cancellation of debt of poorest countries
- Increased aid flows targeted at the poor, children, and health and education sectors
- Support of the UN Convention on the Rights of the Child
- Arms control and support for treaty banning landmines
- Peaceful resolution of conflicts
- Malaria and AIDS vaccines
- Cheaper antiretroviral drugs
- Strengthening of primary health care
- Reduction of marketing of infant formula and 'junk' foods

Individual measures to improve global child health

* Buying locally grown fruit and vegetables reduces use of expensive transport fuel and may increase availability of food for local people in developing countries
* Buying fair trade products directly benefits poor families
* Reducing consumption of fossil fuels conserves the world's resources as well as reducing global warming and its potentially catastrophic effects on developing countries
* Lobbying for remission of debt and increased aid programmes, and individual charitable gifts (especially at times of crisis such as war or environmental catastrophe), can benefit economies and development programmes
* Boycotting multinational corporations which use irresponsible marketing or employ child labour helps reduce these practices

Developing health care services

There is huge variation in the quality, efficiency, and effectiveness of health care systems in developing countries, and some notable examples of good practice in countries which have succeeded in making a major impact on child health and population health generally. Cuba, Kerala in India, and Nicaragua, for example, provide many pointers to the best models of health care. Key elements which contribute to the success of such systems are shown in the box below.

Means of improving health care in developing countries

* Orientate training of doctors towards primary care, community care, and prevention
* Train doctors and other health workers together to promote a multidisciplinary team approach
* Provide inducements for health workers to work in rural areas
* Develop primary and secondary health care as an integrated system
* Develop the skills of nurses as health practitioners (e.g. Thailand trains midwives to be primary care providers in villages)
* Follow WHO guidelines on integrated care
* Make use of appropriate technology (see below)
* Build a local pharmaceutical industry and essential drug list
* Restrict the development of private practice
* Put a strong emphasis on breast-feeding
* Provide contraceptive advice in maternal and child health clinics
* Integrate immunization with other child health services

Appropriate technology

Appropriate technology is that which is appropriate to the needs and resources of the country concerned: affordable, effective, and sustainable. Some examples are given in the box below.

Appropriate technology for health

- Oral rehydration solution rather than intravenous infusion
- Ultrasound rather than CT scanning
- WHO basic radiological system (BRS) rather than whole body scanning
- Generic drugs rather than branded
- 'Kangaroo' baby technique (skin to skin contact) rather than incubator care
- Solar powered refrigerator rather than paraffin
- Growth charts which are home-based rather than clinic-based
- Training traditional birth attendants in safe childbirth rather than hospital delivery

        See Stanfield *et al.* (1991) *Diseases of children in the subtropics and tropics*

Tackling AIDS and HIV

The boxes below summarise actions needed to tackle the global problem of HIV and AIDS.

Actions needed to tackle the global AIDS problem

- The distribution of antiretroviral drugs to the world's poorest people
- The empowerment of women
- The urgent search for an HIV vaccine
- The care and education of children orphaned by AIDS

        Source: *BMJ* (2002) **324**:181–2

Essential components of HIV/AIDS programmes

A: Prevention of new infections

Reduce sexual transmission:

- Awareness and life skills education, especially for young people
- Condom promotion
- STD control, including for commercial sex workers
- Partner notification

Blood safety:

- HIV testing of transfused blood
- Avoid non-essential blood transfusion
- Recruitment of safe donor pool

Interventions to reduce transmission among injecting drug users

Reduce mother to child transmission by use of:

+ Antiretroviral therapy
+ Avoidance of breast-feeding (where safe to do so)—consider replacement feeding or early weaning

B: Surveillance for HIV infections and AIDS

C: Voluntary counselling and testing

D: Mitigation of HIV related disease

+ Rational approach to care for HIV related disease, especially TB
+ Appropriate preventive therapies

E: Mitigating social impact

+ Minimizing stigma: respect for confidentiality, protection against discrimination
+ Care for AIDS orphans

Source: Grant and De Cock (2001)

Improving child health: the role of research

Many improvements in child health in developing countries have arisen from research projects. There is a need for more locally-based research focussed on means of improving health care, perhaps financed by the north.

Areas of research likely to benefit child health

+ Improving vitamin A status through fortification or supplementation
+ Reducing mother to infant transmission of HIV
+ Malaria prevention through use of insecticide-treated bed nets
+ Prevention of accidental injury
+ Prevention of child abuse

Source: *BMJ working Group on Women and Child Health*
(2002) **324**: *1444–7*

Child care for young children

UNICEF has called on governments and international agencies to fund early childhood care fully, from before birth to teenage years, but with a particular emphasis on the ages up to three years. It is estimated that $80bn (£57bn) a year is need to give every newborn in the world a good start in life. UNICEF identified four key points:

1. Early childhood care is a human rights issue. All children are entitled to registration at birth, sound nutrition, health care, clean water, adequate sanitation, basic education, and an opportunity to reach their full potential.

2. Early childhood care is grounded in sound science and practical experience. Comprehensive early care should provide the building blocks for social and intellectual competence.

3. Early childhood care is a solid investment. For every $1 spent on early childhood care there is a $7 return through cost savings, based on studies showing that participants in preschool and day care are less likely to experience illnesses and to drop out of school.

4. The three major challenges are poverty, conflict, and HIV/AIDS. Effective interventions against these challenges would bring major benefit to the health of the world's children.

The UN Convention on the Rights of the Child (UNCRC)

Internationally, the UN Convention on the Rights of the Child is an extremely important means of improving child health and well-being and is a vital tool for advocacy by all those concerned with child public health.

Key principles of the UN Convention on the Rights of the Child

- Best interests of the child to be a primary consideration in legislation
- Rights to survival and development
- Rights to express their views and freedom of expression
- Access to information of benefit and protection from injurious information
- Protection from violence, abuse, and neglect
- Right to the highest attainable standard of health
- Right to an adequate standard of living
- Protection from economic exploitation

Only one country has yet to ratify the convention, namely the USA. Each country which has ratified it has a responsibility to report to the UN Committee on the Rights of the Child in Geneva every five years. This provides a public opportunity to examine a country's record in upholding children's rights. Health care professionals and others concerned with child health and children's rights may join with non-governmental organizations in challenging or supporting the actions taken and the official reports submitted by governments. Enforcement and monitoring of the Convention—at local, national, and international level—is vital, and is an important public health role.

Sustainable development

The final word goes to another concept which has important implications for international child health and in which we are all implicated—that of sustainable development, which 'fulfils the needs of the present generation without endangering the needs of future generations'. Sustainable development should not lead to the production of environmental burdens to be inherited by future generations, such as the build-up of greenhouse gases, pollution of seas and rivers, production of unmanageable amounts of waste, and loss of natural habitats. This means that businesses, governments, and individuals have a duty to conserve and reuse the limited resources of the planet. The rationale for sustainable development is that the human race, through environmental degradation, is immensely damaging to the Earth and must now tackle this huge problem. Examples of depleting resources are in the box below.

Depleted resources

Fisheries: nearly 50% of all fish stocks are fully exploited; 20% are overexploited
Forests: on current trends, by 2025 15% of all forest species will be extinct
Air pollution: 3 million people die each year due to air pollution and 5 million due to unsafe water
Water: most groundwater resources are being depleted at a rate of 0.1–0.5% per year
(Organisation of Economic Co-operation and Development, 2002)

The concept of an 'ecological footprint' is also interesting and useful: it is the area of land required to provide for the needs and absorb the waste of a person, group, city, or business. For example, a family in a developed country who run two 'gas-guzzling' cars, are profligate in their use of energy for heating, lighting, household appliances, and so on, who purchase high proportions of imported food, and generate large amounts of non-recycled waste, will have a large ecological footprint. On the other hand, a similar family who use bicycles and public transport, grow their own food on an allotment, use solar panels for heating, and make maximum use of composting and recycling will have a much smaller ecological footprint.

The footprint of London equals the UK's entire area of productive land—around 125 times London's surface area; a total of 19.7 million hectares. European citizens average a footprint of three hectares each, and North Americans require between four and five. Yet worldwide, only one and a half hectares of productive land is available per person. 'Ecological trespassing' is thus inevitable, with developed countries using up land and resources which properly belong to others.

The implication is that we should all attempt to live within the footprint rightfully available to us, and that consumption and overuse of resources by rich countries should be reduced drastically. The lack of attention paid to sustainable development and ecological trespass affects the health of children across the globe significantly, principally through global warming which is causally related to the burning of fossil fuels. There is no doubt that global warming is taking place and will affect children's health both directly and indirectly. It is very important that all those with an interest in improving children's health support the concept of sustainable development and attempt to live sustainable lifestyles.

Further reading

HIV and AIDS

Grant, A. and De Cock, K. (2001). HIV infection and AIDS in the developing world. *BMJ*; **322**: 1475–8.

Poverty, debt, and health

Benatar, S. (1997). Africa in the twenty-first century: can despair be turned to hope? *BMJ*; **315**:1444–6.

Black, R.E., Morris, S.S., and Bryce, J. (2003). Where and why are 10 million children dying every year? *Lancet*; **361**:2226–343.

BMA (2000). *Debt and health*. British Medical Association, London.

Carnall, D. (1999). Demographic entrapment. *BMJ*; **319**:1012.

Haines, A., Heath, I., and Smith, R. (2000). Joining together to combat poverty. *BMJ*; **320**:1–2.

Haines, A. and Smith, R. (1997). Working together to reduce poverty's damage. *BMJ*; **314**:529.

Working Group on Women and Child Health: F. Dabis, J. Orne–Gliemann, F. Perez, V. Leroy, M.L. Newell, A. Coutsoudis, and H. Coovadia (2002). Improving child health: the role of research *BMJ*; **324**:1444–7.

War and conflict

Plunkett, M.C.B. and Southall, D.P. (1998). War and children. *Archives of Disease in Childhood*; **78**:72–7.

Southall, D.P. and O'Hare, B.A.M. (2002). Empty arms: the effect of the arms trade on mothers and children. *BMJ*; **325**:1457–61.

Asylum seekers

Burnett, A. and Fassil, Y. (2000). *Meeting the needs of asylum seekers and refugees: an information and resource pack for healthcare workers in the UK*. Department of Health, London.

Levenson, R. and Sharma, A. (1999). *The health of refugee children—Guidelines for Paediatricians*. King's Fund and Royal College of Paediatrics and Child Health, London.

Levenson, R. with Coker, N. (1999). *The health of refugees—a guide for GPs*. King's Fund Publishing, London.

Tropical diseases

Stanfield, P., Brueton, M., Chan, M., Parkin, M., and Waterston, T. (ed.) (1991). *Diseases of children in the subtropics and tropics*. Edward Arnold, London.

Other

Hawamdeh, H. and Spencer, N. (2001). Work, family socioeconomic status and growth among working boys in Jordan. *Archives of Disease in Childhood*; **84**:311–14.

Lansdown, G., Waterston, T., and Baum, D. (1996). Implementing the UN Convention on the Rights of the Child in the health service. *BMJ*; **313**:1565–6.

Morley, D. and Lovel, H. (1986). *My name is today*. Macmillan, London.

Trouiller, P., Olliaro, P., Torreele, E., Orbinski, J., Laing, R., and Ford, N. (2002). Drug development for neglected diseases: a deficient market and a public health policy failure. *Lancet*; **359**:2188–94.

UNICEF (yearly). *State of the world's children*. Oxford University Press, Oxford.

Waterston, T., and Lenton, S. (2000). Sustainable development, human-induced climate change and child health. *Arch Dis Child*; **82**:95–7.

Chapter 3

Child public health—lessons from the past

History is important because it can provide explanations for current affairs and also lessons in how things can change. Child health clearly has changed dramatically for the better over the last few centuries, but those who would see further improvements can learn a lot from what has gone before. An awareness of previous mistakes can prevent the same mistakes being made again.

The history of child public health is both the history of children's health and the history of society's response to the health problems and diseases of children. As the health of children is an important indicator of the health of society, the history of child public health is closely related to the history of public health in general. Although some childhood diseases and health problems are caused by specific agents (bacteria, pollutants, or genes) child health is also determined by social and environmental conditions. A historical account of child public health therefore needs to address changes in social policy and in the social and physical environment, as well as trends in disease incidence and prevalence.

Public health initiatives are easier to implement when philanthropic social attitudes prevail. Many of the public health improvements of previous centuries have been underpinned by changing attitudes towards the health and welfare of vulnerable members of society—the poor, the sick, and children. These have driven legislative regulation of child labour and supported the development of public services like universal education and child health services. These philanthropic attitudes have also had an impact on children's health by influencing the care babies and children receive from their parents at home. There have been substantial changes over this period in parenting practices and in what is regarded as a desirable home environment for children.

Public health reforms may also be driven by self interest and by the interests of the state. Many of the improvements to housing and sanitation in poor areas of cities were introduced, at least in part, to protect the rich from infectious disease. The development of school health services following the Boer War was driven, to some extent, by the need for fit young men to serve in the armed forces to protect the interests of the British Empire. These two forces—self interest and philanthropy—while very different philosophically have frequently acted synergistically to bring about change.

Early times: history relates affairs of state, not so much affairs of the home

The historian tracing the history of child health, and the ways in which societies have tried to improve it, needs to access records on the subject of childhood. These, it would appear, are in short supply. The affairs of the home, where women and children spend their days, have been regarded as of lesser importance than the affairs of state, and few written records have been preserved. Victorian archivists appear to have selectively destroyed much that was recorded in women's letters or accounts. Historians, who have tackled the task of understanding family life in the distant past, have therefore worked with snippets of information in records often written for other purposes. Gleaning, collating, and interpreting such information is an arduous task. Some of the texts which are available paint a pretty dismal picture of childhood in the Western World from the late Middle Ages to the beginning of the eighteenth century. The story they tell is, as DeMause in his *History of childhood* relates, one of

> infanticide and abandonment through to neglect, the rigours of swaddling, the purposeful starving, the beatings, the solitary confinement.

Even at the beginning of the eighteenth century only one in four babies born in London survived. DeMause concluded

> the history of childhood is a nightmare from which we have only recently begun to awake. The further back in history one goes, the lower the level of child care, and the more likely children are to be killed abandoned, beaten, terrorised and sexually abused.

The evidence he presents makes it clear that many children did face such problems, although we do not know what proportion. It is also possible that others fared better. Lawrence Stone, in his *Family, sex and marriage 1600–1800*, also documents widespread uncaring attitudes towards babies and children. In the context of such family attitudes, concern for children's health and welfare in social policy and legislation might have seemed quite out of place.

The eighteenth century: the emergence of more humanitarian attitudes

In contrast to material about child care in the home, historians have a wealth of material to work with in the area of social policy. Here they have been able to demonstrate the emergence of more humanitarian attitudes from the eighteenth century onwards, gaining in prominence and breadth up until the present time. These changing attitudes were manifested in legislation regulating child labour and in the establishment of hospitals and health services for poor women and children. At the same time attitudes to vulnerable adults were also softening, resulting in the abolition of slavery and in the extension of the franchise. These developments have been attributed to the endeavours of individual social reformers, such as Thomas Coram, but they could not have achieved the social reforms that they did without the active interest and backing of a broad section of society.

Milestones in child public health 1700–1800

- 1722—Guy's Hospital admits children to women's ward
- 1739—Foundling Hospital in London founded by Thomas Coram
- 1769—Dispensary for Sick Children of the Poor opened in Red Lion Square, London
- 1784—A treatise on the diseases of children, by M. Underwood, published by the Royal College of Surgeons in Ireland, laid the foundations of paediatrics
- 1788—1788 Regulation of Chimney Sweepers and their Apprentices Act required apprentices to be at least eight years old; the Act was not well enforced

In the eighteenth century, most children still lived in the country.

Welfare reforms regulating child labour and the establishment of hospitals and health services improved the lot of some children in cities.

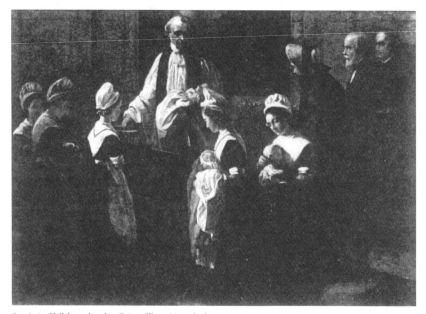

Fig. 3.1 Children in the Foundling Hospital.

The nineteenth century: a time of ups and downs for child health

Philanthropic attitudes were by no means the only driving force in social change and some policy changes during this era were antithetical to child health. For example, the first half of the nineteenth century saw standards of living rise very greatly in the wealthy sectors of the population. At the same time the policy of enclosure of the land had made rural existence precarious for the farm servant, and the agricultural slump following the Napoleonic Wars turned many into paupers. During this period of great need, the 1834 Poor Law aimed to withdraw the 'outdoor relief' which had supported poor families during periods of unemployment, and substituted the draconian provision of the workhouse. In practice this law was not fully implemented and outdoor relief continued for some time.

Changes in the physical environment

Although cities were profoundly unpleasant places to live during the nineteenth century, they provided a greater chance of a livelihood than the countryside. As a result, large numbers of people moved to the cities. In 1800, 20% of the population lived in towns and cities; by 1921 this figure had risen to 80%. Rising city populations meant problems with the distribution of food, and prices were such that the staple diet amongst the poor was bread and tea. There was widespread adulteration of food. A survey in 1841 suggested that only the best paid workers earned enough to achieve an adequate nutritional intake. Both women and children had to work to eat, but the lion's share of the inadequate household food went to the men.

In the middle of the nineteenth century the advent of the railways improved supplies to the cities, bringing in cheap fish and coal. However, widespread adulteration of foodstuffs continued until the beginning of the twentieth century. At the turn of the century Professor Cantlie proclaimed that 'it was impossible to find anybody whose grandfather or grandmother had been born in London'. He suggested that offspring of native Londoners were born so weak and debilitated that 'nature stepped in and denied the continuance of such'.

At the same time as the social policies which allowed these conditions prevailed, there were individuals who were undertaking surveys, establishing hospitals, writing reports on the conditions of the poor, and voicing their concerns in public. Social reformers and public health doctors like Edwin Chadwick, William Duncan, and William Farr argued the need for reforms on the basis of enlightened self interest as well as on the basis of philanthropy. Pointing out that cholera and typhoid from contaminated water supplies were no respecters of social class, they pushed through reforms at national and local level, improving the housing and sanitary conditions of the poor. Social reformers also developed the utilitarian arguments that starving workers were less productive than those who were well fed. From time to time they were able to achieve a sufficient vote in parliament or in the local authorities to achieve the investment or legislation required to improve the lot of children and their families (see Table 3.1).

The 1848 Public Health Act enabled local towns and districts to set up health boards with their own medical officers of health. These new public health doctors supervised the sanitary inspectors, whose job it was to notify and prevent infections diseases and to ensure adequate water supplies. They were well placed to gather and present statistics about epidemics of disease and advance arguments for spending on the infrastructure of the towns and cities. Rural authorities were, however, very

Table 3.1 Milestones in child public health 1800–1900

Date	Event	Effect
1802	Health and Morals of Apprentices Act	Restricted working hours to 12 hours in the daytime, with a requirement for elementary education
1819	Cotton Mills and Factories Act	Prohibited children under nine from working in cotton mills
1831	In the face of cholera epidemics, local Boards of Health established	They were to appoint and oversee district inspectors, to report on sanitary conditions of the poor, and to endeavour to remedy defects
1831 & 1833	Mills and Factory Acts	Introduced compulsory holidays and required two hours a day elementary education for younger children
1833	First children's ward opened in a Hospital (Guy's, London)	
1842	Edwin Chadwick reported on the poor state of sanitation in the country and contrasted life expectancy in different social classes	Report led to the establishment of the Royal Commission for Inquiry into the State of Towns and Populous Cities
1847	First Medical Officer of Health Appointed in Liverpool (William Duncan)	
1848	Public Health Act	Created Central Board of Health and required permanent local Boards of Health to be set up outside London
1852	Royal Hospital for Sick Children, Great Ormond Street, founded	
1858	Mines and Collieries Act	Prohibited employment underground of children under 10
1862	Manchester and Salford Ladies Health Society appointed the first health visitors	These visitors 'being women of working class to visit the poor and teach them the rules of health and child care'.
1867	Vaccination Act (later rescinded)	Made vaccination with cow pox compulsory for all infants
1870	Education Act	Attempted to provide elementary education for all children; many local school boards did not use their powers to compel children to attend
1872	Infant Life Protection Act	Required all those who took in two or more children for reward to be registered

Table 3.1 (continued)

Date	Event	Effect
1874	Births and Deaths Registration Act	Introduced a penalty for failure to notify and required medical certificate of cause of death
1875	Public Health Act	Consolidated and amended previous Acts; empowered local authorities to provide hospitals and medicines and medical assistance to the poor
1876	Elementary Education Act	Placed a duty on parents to ensure that their children received elementary education
1889	Prevention of Cruelty to and Protection of Children Act	Ill treatment and neglect to be punishable by law
1893	Education Act	
1899	First Infant Welfare Centre opened in St Helen's	
1900	First free milk supplied to nursing mothers	

reluctant to make such appointments, knowing that they were likely to result in increased expenditure on sanitation and isolation hospitals. It was not until 1910 that the Town and Housing Act made medical officer of health appointments compulsory. It was recognized that the new public health doctors were likely to make themselves unpopular with the wealthy burghers who dominated the committees of the county councils, and their appointments were protected by a measure of independence. They could not be dismissed from their posts by a decision of the local authorities alone. In theory therefore, they were free to speak out about health and social problems, making the case for reform. While many did do so and, in this way, contributed to important improvements in the living conditions of the poor, many others kowtowed to prevalent 'victim blaming' attitudes which were used to justify lack of investment in health infrastructure.

The history of child public health has thus been dictated by ebbs and flows. Against a backdrop of gradual progress there have been many setbacks. Powerful advocates have needed to gather data, establish alliances, and make the case for reform. They would often be opposed by those who saw no need to change the status quo and might bear the brunt of the financial consequences of reform.

Changes in child care practices among the wealthy

Such records as do exist suggest that life for many children in the nineteenth century was a definite improvement on life in the eighteenth. The practice of swaddling

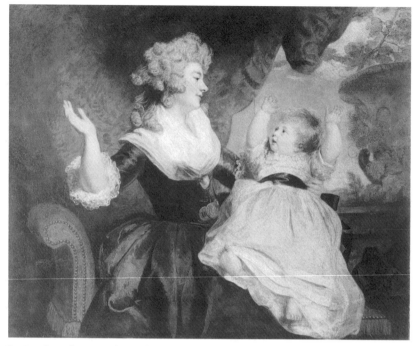

Fig. 3.2 Georgiana, Duchess of Devonshire, set a new trend when she chose, in 1783, to breast-feed her own daughter. (Devonshire Collection, Chatsworth. Reproduced by permission of the Duke of Devonshire and the Chatsworth Settlement Trustees. Photograph: Photographic Survey, Courtauld Institute of Art.)

(which renders babies passive, quiet, and easy to care for) had largely been abandoned during the eighteenth century. The practice, amongst the wealthy, of putting children out to wet nurses began to disappear when Georgiana, Duchess of Devonshire, an influential trend-setter of her time, elected in 1783 to breast-feed her own daughter (Fig. 3.2).

Although boarding schools developed and flourished in this era, the younger children of the rich came to be cared for in their own homes by mothers or servants. They seem to have been beaten and whipped less frequently, but it was still common during the nineteenth century for small children to be punished with food restriction or to be shut in dark closets for long periods.

Child care amongst the poor

The life of most children in the labouring classes continued to be grim. Mothers needed to work up to and straight after childbirth to bring in sufficient income, but the industrial revolution had separated the world of work from the world of the home, so children were often abandoned to the care of someone else from a very young age. Maternal mortality was high, so many children were brought up in motherless households. Babies were frequently fed gin and narcotics to allay their fretfulness for want of food. Many children thus grew up supervised by children little

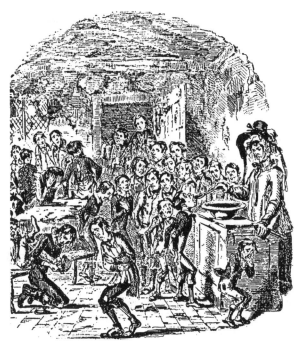

Fig. 3.3 Cartoon of Dotheboys Hall. The writings of Charles Dickens in the 1830s and 1840s have provided an enduring image of life in boarding schools during that period. (Source: Charles Dickens, *The life and adventures of Nicholas Nickleby* (1987). Oxford University Press, Oxford.)

older than themselves, in a hazardous environment, fed on inadequate quantities of bread and tea, and frequently abused. Their survival was rewarded with a move into the relentless, monotonous, and dangerous world of factory work at the age of six or seven. The Education Act in 1870, and several subsequent Acts, attempted to establish universal elementary education, but it was some time before these Acts took effect.

In the nineteenth century

- The populations of cities grew dramatically and conditions deteriorated.
- Sanitation was poor, food prices high, foodstuffs adulterated, and child labour the norm.
- The practice among the rich of putting babies out to wet nurses disappeared, but children were still sent away to boarding school at young ages.
- A series of cholera outbreaks led to a number of sanitary reforms and the gradual establishment of effective sanitation and public health services.
- A series of Education Acts aimed to establish universal elementary education, but they did not take effect for some time.
- Childhood mortality rates started to fall in the latter half of the century.

The twentieth century: interest in child public health waxes and wanes

Although the medical profession played a role in advocating and enabling change, the improvements in child public health which occurred in the eighteenth and nineteenth centuries were achieved almost entirely through changes to the social and environmental conditions in which children lived. During the twentieth century, particularly the latter half, public health was also informed by advances in understanding of the causes of disease and the development of medical practice. Indeed, public health practice became increasingly dominated by the provision of medical services and by attempts to prevent or treat specific diseases and conditions.

The emergence of epidemiology

By the beginning of the twentieth century, routine monitoring of death rates in different age groups and from different causes was practical and the discipline of epidemiology developed. It was possible to demonstrate quantitative improvements in public health by charting reductions in mortality rates. Figure 3.4 shows the mortality rates amongst males in three age groups—under 1 year of age, 1–4 years of age, and 5–14 years (rates in girls are very similar). The data are presented as a logarithmic plot which allows changes in the very different rates in the three groups to be compared on the same graph. The graph shows rates to be falling amongst older children from 1850 onwards and those in 1–4 year olds from 1870. Infant death rates however remained high, only beginning to fall in 1905.

Services to reduce infant mortality

These infant mortality rates, resistant as they appeared to be to the social and environmental improvements to which falling mortality rates in older children were

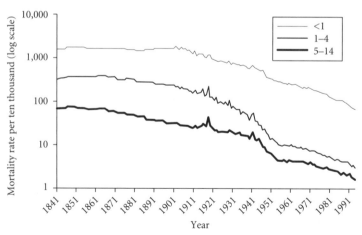

Fig. 3.4 Male childhood mortality rates in England and Wales 1841–1991. (Drawn from data provided by Dr John Charlton, Office for National Statistics, London by SSB.)

attributed, were a cause of concern. Public health interest therefore focussed on reducing the common causes of infant deaths as recorded on death certificates— infection, poor nutrition, and 'overlaying'.

There was much discussion about the ignorance and fecklessness of mothers. Charitable societies were the first to develop services to support mothers, paying for midwives, health visitors, and infant welfare centres. Charitable provision continued to be an important source of health care for the poor throughout the first half of the twentieth century. Subsequently, some local authorities also started to develop preventive services, appointing community health doctors and midwives.

Several Medical Officers of Health and many of those involved in the local charitable societies suggested that the social and physical environment—inadequate nutrition, sickness, overwork, insanitary housing, and overcrowding—were more to blame for high infant mortality rates than was the knowledge of mothers. They made the case for the provision of monetary benefits to mothers, and provided them with free milk and meals in infant welfare centres. There was, however, a reluctance at national level to accept that poverty was the key problem and public health policy and local authority provision continued to concentrate on services to 'educate' mothers.

> Services were established first by local charitable societies, and subsequently by local authorities, to educate mothers about the proper way to look after babies. In order to avail themselves of these services many mothers would have had to run the gauntlet of patronizing advice and disapproval of a lifestyle over which they had little control.

From 1905 onwards, infant mortality rates started to fall. Whether this change could be attributed entirely to the new child public health services is doubtful. However, the public health doctors of the day were quick to claim that this was the case. Maternal mortality rates, however, continued to give cause for concern. These concerns led to the passing of the Maternity and Child Welfare Act (1918) which required local authorities to appoint a committee 'to be concerned with the health of expectant and nursing mothers and of children under 5 years' and encouraged the development of infant welfare clinics and health visiting. For mothers this Act was a mixed blessing. The availability of health care free of the stigma of the Poor Law, the provision of milk and food to mothers, and the setting up of child health surveillance programmes are likely to have made a valuable contribution to mothers' and children's health. However, in order to avail themselves of these services many mothers would have had to run the gauntlet of patronizing advice and disapproval of a lifestyle over which they had little control.

Some of the advice which was provided to mothers by health professionals during the early part of the twentieth century went beyond that designed to improve nutrition and reduce infection. In 1921, the Society for the Health of Women and

Children published the child care manual of the paediatrician Truby King. This advised mothers: In the interests of their babies' health and welfare, to feed them by the clock, to ensure that their bowels moved every morning, to avoid fond and foolish overindulgence and spoiling (said to be more damaging than intentional cruelty or callous neglect), and to note that 'obedience in infancy is the foundation for all later powers of self control'. This advice, as can be seen in Chapter 5, had a pervasive and detrimental effect on the nurture of babies in the UK and their mental and physical health in later life.

School health services

The Boer War (1899–1902) played an interesting part in the development of twentieth-century child health services. The low level of fitness amongst recruits to the armed forces in this war so alarmed the establishment that an Interdepartmental Committee on Physical Deterioration was established to investigate the health of school children. The Committee heard evidence from teachers, school inspectors, and local public health doctors, which suggested that a high proportion of children were undernourished and suffering from recurrent illness, to the extent that they could not benefit from education. There was increasing concern about the health of the urban poor and discussion about whether this was improving or declining.

> The low level of fitness of recruits to the armed forces in the Boer War led to a health survey of school children which showed a high proportion of children to be undernourished and suffering from recurrent illness.

The report of this Committee in 1904 made recommendations on a wide spectrum of health matters, many of which were incorporated into health and education legislation in 1907 and 1918. Recommendations included the establishment of the school health service, appointment of health visitors and full-time medical officers in every local authority, periodic medical examination of all school children, health education classes in schools, and the provision of school meals.

The 1907 Act made no provision for children found during inspections to be in need of treatment, and few families had the money to pay for this. Lucky children lived in cities where charitable hospitals or dispensaries made some provision for the treatment of children, either through subscriptions schemes or private donations, but rural children fared less well. The 1918 Education Act enabled, but did not require local authorities to offer free treatment for defects found. Local authorities varied in the alacrity with which they availed themselves of this opportunity to spend local taxes. The provision of free school meals, which legislation permitted but did not require, was similarly patchy. Thus, while the legislation which enabled the development of the school health service marks an important milestone in the history of child public health, it did not necessarily improve the lot of children throughout the country. Indeed for many it meant little more than the requirement to submit to somewhat unpleasant medical inspections and enforced delousing.

School medical inspections did, however, make a contribution to epidemiology, providing the first statistics on the level of disease in living populations, and many believed that they made an important contribution to child health. By the time of the Second World war, some Directors of Public Health were claiming that

> the child of 1938–9 was bigger, more resistant to disease, better nourished, cleaner and in every way fitter to bear the strain of wartime than his predecessor in 1914 and much of the credit for this can be unhesitatingly given to the school health service.
> Dr J. Alison Glover in Chadwick lecture, May 1942.

Others, however, noted that all was not yet quite perfect.

> The evacuation of our cities and the findings of our Medical Recruitment Boards have laid bare such a mass of preventable disability that we are ashamed.
> Ministry of Health Hospital Survey, the hospital services of Berkshire, Buckinghamshire, Oxfordshire HMSO 1954.

The years of the Second World War, with the introduction of rationing and high rates of employment, were widely regarded as good for children's health. Growth rates continued to rise and dental health showed a marked improvement.

In the first half of the twentieth century

- Public health interest focussed on infant and maternal mortality rates and led to the setting up of maternal and infant welfare services by charitable organizations and city public health departments.
- Although many believed that the poor health of mothers and infants was attributable to poverty, public health officials blamed the fecklessness and ignorance of mothers.
- Recruitment for the Boer War led to recognition of the high levels of disability and disease among children.
- The school meals and school health services were established, and regular statistics on levels of disease were generated by medical inspections.

Declining interest in child public health

Around the beginning of the twentieth century, public health policy was informed by the belief that health in childhood plays an important part in determining health in adulthood. This belief led public health officials to anticipate a drop in adult mortality rates commensurate with the improvement in childhood mortality rates that had occurred at the end of the nineteenth century. Figure 3.5 contrasts the continuing decline in mortality rates in 1–4 and 5–15 year olds from 1870 to 1950 with the relatively constant mortality rate in the same generations as adults. It shows that people who were born at the end of the nineteenth century experienced lower childhood mortality rates than those born earlier, but that mortality rates in this generation (age 55–64 years) did not show a decline to the extent which was expected in the

Table 3.2 Milestones in child public health 1900–50

Date	Event	Effect
1904	Report of the Interdepartmental Committee on Physical Deterioration	Recommended a wide range of public health measures which were gradually implemented over the next 50 years, including: establishment of the school health service, appointment of full-time medical officers of health and health visitors in every local authority, medical inspections and health education classes in schools, provision of free school meals, registration of stillbirths
1907	Education Act	Local authorities given duty to inspect and attend health of children at elementary schools
1908	Children Act	Gave powers for the removal of children from undesirable situations and placing children in care
1915	Compulsory birth notification by midwives to medical officers of health introduced	
1918	Maternal and Child Welfare Act	Required local authorities to appoint committees to be concerned with maternity and child welfare, and suggested full-time health visitors, free hospital care for complicated pregnancies, and maternal and child welfare clinics up to five years
1918	Education Act	Raised school leaving age to 14 years (not implemented immediately) and abolished elementary school fees school
1921	Diptheria antitoxin used to protect children	
1927	Tetanus toxoid and BCG vaccine first introduced	
1928	British Paediatric Association founded	
1929	Abolition of the Poor Law and conversion of workhouses into hospitals	

Table 3.2 (continued)

Date	Event	Effect
1944	Education Act	Secondary education to be provided free for all children (1947 Act— up to 15 years; 1973 Act—up to 16 years); free milk, subsidized meals, and free medical and dental inspection; special education for handicapped children
1947	National Health Service Act	
1948	Universal Family Allowance introduced	

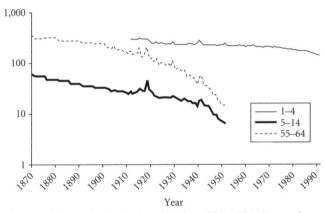

Fig. 3.5 Male mortality rate in England and Wales 1870–1991. Drawn from data provided by Dr John Charlton, Office for National Statistics, London.

period 1925–1975. Death rates in this age group only began to decline from 1970 onwards.

These observations seem to have alarmed public health officials of the time and led to speculation about the cause. The theories of eugenicists such as Karl Pearson, who believed that the public health reforms were leading to the survival of 'degenerate and enfeebled stock' seemed to some to offer an attractive explanation of the unexpected trends. Statistics showing an increase in deaths due to cancer and heart disease fuelled the belief that these new epidemics were indeed caused by survival of 'degenerate stock' as a result of the new public health services for mothers and children.

The impact and aftermath of the First World War and the depression of the 1930s are likely to have contributed to the static adult mortality rates in that era, but do not seem to have been considered a sufficient cause. Instead, the juxtaposition of these relatively static adult mortality rates in a generation for whom childhood mortality rates suggested greatly improved childhood health, together with apparent epidemics of heart disease and cancer, seem to have led public health officials to discard theories relating adult health to child health, and to focus on contemporary causes of disease. The epidemic of heart disease appeared at the time to be more of a problem in those from the upper social classes than the lower social classes, diverting attention away from the social environment as a cause.

The middle of the twentieth century therefore saw a shift in focus of public health research and policy away from concerns with child health, the assumption being made that any gains to public health which could be achieved through improving child health had already been achieved. Demonstration of the critical role that smoking played in the development of lung cancer and subsequently heart disease must have fuelled the belief that adult lifestyle was the field in which solutions to contemporary public health problems were to be found.

The establishment of the NHS in 1948 led to an increasing interest in the treatment of illness in adults. As a result child public health more or less disappeared from the research agenda of those practicing in the new medical specialty of public health. Policy developments in public health concentrated on encouraging adults to adopt healthy lifestyles and, subsequently, on the early identification and treatment of disease through screening. The policy developments with an impact on child public health which did occur during this period, for example in child protection, were largely driven from outside public health. Child public health became the concern of community child health doctors and health visitors.

With the 1974 local government and NHS reorganization these services were transferred to the NHS, and with NHS reorganizations in 1990 and 1997, from health authorities to general practice. The 1974 reorganization saw the abolition of the post of Medical Officer of Health and the separation of medical public health from community child health services. Although for a decade expertise in child public health continued to be provided by consultants in public health at area health authority level, further NHS reforms and developments in the medical specialty of public health have resulted in less and less expertise in child public health amongst doctors trained in public health.

The low professional status of community child health doctors and the poor academic base for the specialty meant that they had little influence on the development of policy. Although there have been attempts to restate the importance of community child health services—for example, the Court Report in 1974—they had only a limited impact at the time. A delayed effect was the establishment of the medical specialty of community paediatrics, the appointment of consultant community paediatricians, and the establishment of university departments of community child health. These changes are now having a gradual impact on the status of community child health services and on research and development in child public health.

Vaccination and immunization

Although this was an inactive period, in terms of child health policy, child health itself witnessed great advances as a result of the introduction of new vaccinations and immunizations. Childhood vaccination has a long history, but most important developments took place in the twentieth century. (The first Vaccination Act of 1867, which was never fully implemented and was later withdrawn, made vaccination of children against smallpox compulsory.) The interwar period witnessed the development and introduction of vaccines against the toxin produced by diphtheria and tetanus and against tuberculosis. In the 1950s, vaccines were developed against polio and pertussis and introduced nationwide. BCG vaccination was offered to all school leavers. Measles vaccination was introduced in 1968, rubella vaccination of school girls in 1970, and the combined measles, mumps, rubella vaccine to one-year-olds in1988. The last decade has witnesses the introduction of two further vaccines, one against Haemophilus influenza and one against meningitis C. Together these vaccines have played a part in the dramatic reduction in health problems attributable to infectious diseases in childhood.

Screening programmes

The second area of practice development in twentieth century child health has been in the development of screening programmes, Childhood screening programmes evolved from the routine medical inspections required for all school children by the 1918 Education Act. The inspection of preschool children in child health clinics with the aim of identifying those likely to need special education followed. These programmes were not screening programmes in the sense in which the term is now used, but they did identify children with health needs which were not being met and were able to provide treatment for some problems. It was, however, not until the establishment of the NHS and the medical specialties of paediatrics, ear, nose, and throat surgery, and ophthamology that these childhood screening programmes really took off. By the 1980s a very large number of children were being referred to these services for treatment of minor childhood illnesses and developmental abnormalities (e.g. glue ear, tonsillitis, amblyopia).

A national standard programme of child health surveillance and monitoring has now been recommended for both child health and school health.

In the late 1980s, paediatricians and public health specialists working in community child health started to examine the benefits of such programmes and suggested that some were resulting in overtreatment. (See Chapter 4 for information on the evaluation of screening programmes.) Some of the programmes offered to parents and children in the 1980s were raising parental concerns about problems which were likely to resolve spontaneously and for which no useful intervention could be offered. A series of reports from these Committees—the Hall Reports—identified the components of these programmes which are beneficial and recommended the discontinuation of those which were not. A national standard programme of child health surveillance and monitoring has now been recommended and endorsed by a new National Screening Committee for both child health and school health.

Many of the current screening tests such as physical examination for developmental hip (acetabular) dysplasia or congenital heart disease, and vision, hearing, and developmental screening remain under much scrutiny. The imprecision of the screening tests, bringing with it problems associated with false positive and false negative results, and uncertainty about the extent of benefit from treatment, mean that it is difficult to demonstrate that overall these programmes do more good than harm. Other programmes—antenatal screening for spina bifida and Down's syndrome, neonatal screening for phenylketonuria—have had an important impact on the incidence of disability attributable to these health problems.

> In the late twentieth century there was a lack of interest in child public health. Hospital and health services for children continued to be developed but public health services concentrated on adults.

The development of hospital paediatric services

Until the twentieth century, sick people who could afford to do so were looked after in their homes. Lying in hospitals (maternity), hospitals for the mentally ill, for foundlings, and for people who were dying had been built in the eighteenth century on charitable donations, but provision was patchy and these were dangerous places. Until Semmelweiss and Nightingale identified measures to control the spread of infection in the mid nineteenth century, mortality was very high. In the second half of the nineteenth century, concerns about the spread of infectious diseases led to the establishment by local authorities of municipal hospitals, separate from workhouses, and by 1911 there were over 1000 of these hospitals. Children suffering from diphtheria and other infectious diseases would be sent to such hospitals, where they existed. In areas where they did not exist, the diagnosis of a case of diptheria would usually herald the closure of the local school and the suspension of education until the epidemic had past.

In 1921, the newly established Ministry of Health recommended that hospitals should be overseen by a Hospital's Commission and should receive a block grant from Parliament in addition to their charitable funding. This was the beginning of a national hospital service and the rapid development of effective medical care. With the abolition of the Poor Law in 1929, large numbers of workhouses were turned into hospitals and hospital stock increased. The establishment of the NHS in 1947 accelerated the process. Although the Royal College of Surgeons in Ireland had published *A treatise on the diseases of children* in 1784, laying the foundation for the establishment of the speciality of paediatrics, training of paediatric doctors and nurses did not begin until 1931 in Edinburgh—somewhat later than in other European countries. Special medical services for children began to be developed

Table 3.3 Milestones in child public health 1950–99

Date	Event	Effect
1957	Universal immunization with Salk polio vaccine recommended	
1966	Measles vaccine became available	
1970	Rubella immunization available	
1971	Faculty of Community Medicine established (became Faculty of Public Health Medicine in 1989 and Faculty of Public Health in 2003)	
1974	Local government and NHS reorganization	Local authority child health services to be provided by the NHS; NHS organized into regional area and district authorities; post of Medical Officer of Health abolished; community physician posts introduced into NHS
1976	Court Report, 'Fit for the Future' published	
1980	Abolition of area health authorities	
1983	Griffiths Report on the NHS	Recommends general management at every level of the NHS and major cost improvement programmes and commercial orientation introduced
1988	Measles, mumps, rubella vaccine introduced	
1989	Children Act	Provided a radical reform of the law on children; abolished concepts of custody and access; brought in notions of parental responsibility and rights of children to be heard
1990	NHS Act	Established the purchaser-provided split in which health authorities purchased health care from hospital trusts; enabled general practice fundholding
1997	The New NHS—Modern and Dependable	Enables the development of primary care trusts and the abolition of health authorities
1998	Establishment of the Royal College of Paediatrics and Child Health	
1999	Vaccination against Haemophilus influenza introduced	

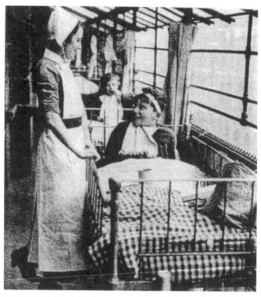

Fig. 3.6 In the 1930s, fresh air treatment on the balcony (Hospital for Sick Children, Great Ormond Street).

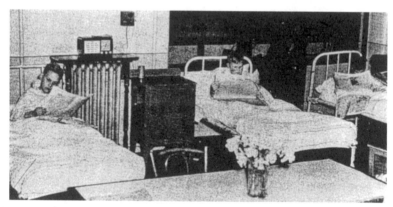

Fig. 3.7 In the 1950s the wards were sparsely furnished and children were arranged tidily in bed in pyjamas for the consultant's ward round (St James' Hospital, Leeds, permission sought).

widely from 1945 onwards. Antibiotics were introduced in 1936, and surgery and anaesthetics gradually became safer.

By the 1960s, surgery on children was commonplace, and a high proportion were hospitalized for tonsillectomy and adenoidectomy. As obstetric care became safer and more sophisticated, more and more babies started to be born in hospital.

Paediatricians began to research the newborn and develop ways of supporting babies born preterm. Successful treatments for childhood cancer were identified.

These advances have made an important contribution to children's health, but as with so many important advances in health care the story is not one of unmitigated success. In the middle of the century, children who were sick with rheumatic fever, TB, renal disease, or Perthe's disease were hospitalized for very long periods of time in strictly regimented wards with very little visiting from their parents, leaving, for many, long-lasting emotional scars. Children with mental and physical disabilities were incarcerated in hospitals where they lived under very cramped conditions, with no privacy and no access to the outdoors. More and more severely preterm babies survived, but many had disabilities. In the 1950s, paediatricians started to recommend, on what turned out to be spurious bases, that all babies should be nursed prone, causing, as can be seen in Fig. 3.8, a 20-year epidemic of death.

Some of these problems have now been rectified—the time children spend in hospital and away from their families is now kept to a minimum; children with disabilities are now cared for in their own homes or in the homes of foster parents, with support from the government; and public education campaigns have ensured that few babies are now nursed prone.

Changes in child care in the twentieth century

Lack of interest in children's health amongst policy makers was accompanied by remarkable changes in child care in the home during the late twentieth century. The practices recommended by Truby King and adopted by many parents have now been largely discontinued, fuelled in part by the research of the paediatricians, John Bowlby and Donald Winnicott, and also by the books of Benjamin Spock and, subsequently, by those of Penelope Leach. A much more nurturing attitude now prevails in most families. The majority of parents also take very seriously their role of stimulating children's cognitive, social, and physical development, and devote time and energy to this. At the same time, dramatic increases in the number of married women in paid employment has meant that babies and children now spend much of their early life outside the home in nurseries and preschool educational facilities.

Parents have also had an effect on children's social and educational environment in other ways. Collectively in the 1960s and 70s, through charitable organizations such as the Preschool Playgroups Association, parents developed a network of inexpensive preschool playgroups which by the late 1980s was supporting the social and educational development of 80% of the country's children. Now, in a similar social movement, parents are disseminating to other parents the implications of research on the impact of common parental practices on children's mental and social health. Through parenting education and support parents are helping each other to learn new ways of responding to children's distress and difficult behaviour, and abandoning unhelpful practices such as physical punishment.

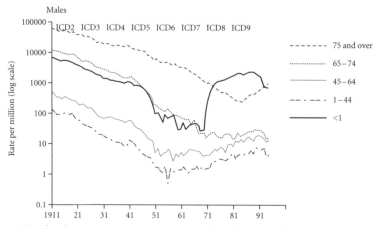

Fig. 3.8 Deaths due to symptoms, signs, and ill-defined conditions. Cot death is the commonest cause of this group of deaths in infancy.
(Source: From Charlton, J. and Murphy, M. The Health of Adult Britain in 1847–1994. ONS 1997, Stationery Office, London.)

The rediscovery of child public health

Although the lack of interest in child public health at academic and policy level during the last fifty years has had a detrimental effect on research and development, a small number of multidisciplinary academic groups have continued to take an interest in child health and in the impact of early life experiences on adult health. The setting up of cohort studies such as the 1000 families study in Newcastle-upon-Tyne in 1947 and the National Birth Cohort Studies in 1946, 1958, 1970, and 2001 are witness to lasting interest in child health. These studies have continued to point to the social and environmental causes of illness and disease in childhood and to provide evidence on the influence of child health on health in adulthood. As a result there is now a large body of literature attesting to the importance of child health and pointing to approaches to improvement.

At the same time, public health research on the impact of health related lifestyles on health has failed to explain the pervasive influence of social inequalities on the most common health problems of adulthood—heart disease and cancer. As can be seen in Chapter 5, the child health literature appears to hold many of the answers, and public health interest in child health is now being rekindled. This, together with the election of a government which espoused somewhat more philanthropic social attitudes than those of governments at the end of the twentieth century, has brought about a resurgence of interest both in social inequalities and in child public health.

There is now a large body of literature attesting to the vital importance of child health and pointing to approaches to improvement. As a result public health interest in child health is now being rekindled.

Some of the child health problems of today are similar to those of the past—for example, the general susceptibility to ill health attributable to living in poverty and inadequate or inappropriate nutrition—but, as Chapter 2 makes clear, many are different. The key problems are now mental health, delinquency and violence, obesity, substance misuse, injuries, asthma, and lack of exercise. Child health is also threatened by the pervasive influence of television, advertising, and marketing, the influence of globalization, and the threat of environmental deterioration. These are important for public health in general, but are especially important for children because of their increased susceptibility and their future expectations of life.

Later in the twentieth century

- Public health officials focussed more on preventing the new epidemics of cancer and heart disease in adults than reducing infant mortality.
- Public health interest in child health declined and child health services were transferred to the NHS
- Attempts to restate the importance of community child health services, such as the Court Report in 1976, had a limited impact.
- Vaccination and immunization services developed and had a dramatic effect on childhood infectious disease rates.
- Preschool child health surveillance services were developed and hospital services for children flourished. These services contributed significantly to child health, but created some unforeseen problems.
- Interest in child public health and addressing social inequalities have recently been rekindled.

Reflections from the past and lessons for child public health practice today

Approaches to the practice of child public health have also changed. It is now rarely important for those practicing public health to know a great deal about drains. On the other hand, the ability to make use of information technology is a key skill. Many of the approaches pertinent in the past remain, however, and as Chapter 2 makes clear, are still important today. One of these is the need to develop long time-scales. Although over this period of history there have been dramatic improvements in child public health, the process has not been one of consistent improvement, but rather of ebbs and flows. There will have been times when it seemed as though things were getting worse. The recommendations of the Report of the Committee on Physical Deterioration took almost 50 years to be implemented. In the end, however, persistence has paid off.

Leadership and advocacy is still very important in bringing about change. However, the leaders of the past who had a special influence could not have achieved what they did without widespread support. Developing alliances between different professional groups and with charitable organizations, and gaining the support of the public is still necessary for success in the long term.

Information is a vital adjunct to advocacy and can clearly influence attitudes. The gathering and presentation of epidemiological data has played an important part in bringing about child health reforms. But the gathering of quantitative data is not enough to improve health. These data can identify the problems but not necessarily the solutions, and solutions developed in the absence of insight from those with the problem can go disastrously wrong. In order to avoid some of the mistakes made around the turn of the last century, the development of solutions to child public health problems needs to involve parents and children, and data need to be gathered by both qualitative as well as quantitative methods. It is also important for those practicing child public health to bear in mind the possibility that the well intentioned interventions they have introduced could be doing more harm than good, and to continually review what they are providing and why.

Child health remains critically dependent on parents and what they are able to provide for their children. Very major changes in the way parents care for children have taken place over the last three centuries and these have played a very important part in improvements in child health. Health professionals have clearly demonstrated that they can have an influence over the way babies are cared for, but some of their interventions have been unhelpful. Enabling parents to support their children's health and development is an important but not an easy task, and it needs to be undertaken in partnership with parents. In Chapter 7 we explore a number of ways in which this can be achieved using lessons from the past together with current insights into the origins of child health and well-being.

Key messages from the past for practice today

- Some aspects of child public health practice have changed greatly, but many remain the same
- Leadership and advocacy is still important
- Patience and long time-scales are essential
- Epidemiological information is vital and influential
- Child health remains critically dependent on parents, and supporting parents remains a key task for those concerned with child public health

Further reading

Bowlby, J. (1953). *Childcare and the growth of love*. Penguin Books Limited, Harmonsworth, Middlesex.

Charlton, J. and Murphy, M. (1997). *The health of adult Britain 1841–1994. Volume 1*. Office of National Statistics. The Stationery Office, London.

Cosler, R. (1992). *In the name of the child: Health and welfare 1880–1940*. Routledge, London.

DeMause, L. (1976). *The history of childhood*. Souvenir Press (Educational and Academic) Ltd, London.

Field, K. (2001). *'Children of the nation?' A study of the health and well-being of Oxfordshire children 1891–1939.* DPhil Thesis, University of Oxford.

Fit for the future: the Committee on Child Health Services Court Report. (Chairman S.D.M. Court) (1976). HMSO, London.

Harris, B. (1995). *The health of the school child: a history of the school medical service in England and Wales.* Open University Press, Buckingham.

King, T.T. (1821). *Feeding and care of baby.* Macmillan, London.

Kuh, D. and Davey Smith, G. (1997). The life course approach: an historical perspective with particular reference to coronary heart disease. In *A life course approach to chronic disease epidemiology* (eds. Kuh, D. and Ben–Schlomo, Y.). Oxford University Press, Oxford.

Leach, P. (1978). *Babyhood. Infant development from birth to two years.* Leach. Penelope.

Leach, P. (1979). *Baby and child.* Photography by Camilla Jessel Leach. Penelope.

Lewis, J. (1980). *The politics of motherhood. Child and maternal welfare in England 1900–1939.* Croom Helm, London.

Spock, B.M. (1955). *Baby and child care.* Bodley Head, London.

Stone, L. (1997). *Family, sex, and marriage 1600–1800.* Weiderfeld & Nicholson, London.

Warren, M.D. (2000). *A chronology of state medicine. Public health, welfare and related services in Britain, 1066–1999.* Faculty of Public Health Medicine, London.

Winnicott, D.Y. (1965). *The family and individual development.* Tavistock Publications, London.

Winnicott, D.Y. (1965). *The maturational processes and the facilitating environment. Studies in the theory of emotional development.* Hogarth Press; Institute of Psycho-Analysis, London.

Winnicott, D.Y. (1975). *Through paediatrics to psychoanalysis.* Hogarth Press; Institute of Psycho-Analysis, London.

Chapter 4

Key concepts and definitions

In this chapter, we present a number of ideas which we have personally found useful in our exploration of child public health. It is by no means an exhaustive list of concepts and definitions; some will be more familiar than others, depending on the reader's own knowledge and background. In many areas there are whole textbooks covering a subject, and signposts to relevant reading are provided.

Health and disease

What is health?

Health is a complex phenomenon: the question of what it is, and how it can be defined, has been much debated over the years by both health professionals and social scientists. The traditional interpretation of the medical establishment was that health was simply the lack of disease—the so-called 'deficit model', which dichotomizes health and disease as opposing and mutually exclusive states and fails to acknowledge any positive aspects of health. The best known attempt to redress the shortcomings of this definition is the World Health Organisation (WHO) definition of health.

> The WHO defines health as 'a state of complete physical, mental and social well-being and not merely the absence of disease or infirmity'.

This definition has been criticized for being over-idealistic and unattainable. Clearly, different models are appropriate for different purposes. In dealing with an outbreak of measles it may be appropriate to consider as healthy those who have avoided that particular disease, but in seeking to promote optimal health within a population such a definition is clearly too limited, and it is important to adopt a wider interpretation which embraces the notion of well-being and includes different dimensions of health.

Another approach involves identifying the factors which influence or contribute to health. For example, Lalonde's 'health field' concept, first described in 1974, recognizes health as being a function of individual lifestyle and the environment, as well as being influenced by human biology and health care provision. This model was used implicitly by the UK government in the 1999 White Paper *Saving Lives: Our Healthier Nation* as the basis for action to promote health.

Health can also be seen in functional terms. The Ottawa Charter for Health Promotion in 1986 produced the following definition:

'Health is a resource for living, not the object of living. It is a positive concept emphasising social and personal resources as well as physical capabilities'.

This perspective was also evident in the resolution of the 30th World Health Assembly at Alma Ata in 1977 which declared that:

> The main social target of governments and of the World Health Organisation in the coming decades should be the attainment by all citizens of the world...of a level of health that will permit them to lead socially and economically productive lives.

In this context, health is considered as a resource for living, which in turn requires certain conditions to ensure its maintenance. These were defined in the Ottawa Charter as:

- Peace
- Shelter
- Education
- Food
- Income
- Stable ecosystem
- Sustainable resources
- Social justice
- Equity

Thus we have the perspective from major organizations. What about that of the general population? Blaxter sought the views of ordinary people about what health meant to them. The answers fell into ten main groups, reflecting the different definitions of health discussed above:

1. Don't know or don't think about it—only know what illness is
2. Health as 'not ill'—lack of symptoms; never having to see the doctor
3. Health as the absence of disease or being well despite disease
4. Health as a reserve—recovering quickly or taking risks and not suffering the effects
5. Health as behaviour—the 'healthy life' (no smoking, no drinking, etc.)
6. Health as physical fitness or athletic prowess
7. Health as energy and vitality
8. Health in terms of social relationships—ability to help and support others
9. Health as function—ability to do things
10. Health as psychosocial well-being—a holistic view of health as 'a state of mind'

But health is also a culturally-determined phenomenon: it is likely that different answers would be obtained if Blaxter's research was repeated in different countries.

Social anthropologists have provided some insight into perceptions of health and the way these relate to perceptions of society, in a range of cultures.

In a book on child public health, it is also important to consider what children think health is. A recent research project in Oxford found that children defined health and well-being in both physical and mental terms. The aspects they described included:

- Being myself
- Absence of illness
- Body working well
- Behaviours that promote health (e.g. cleaning teeth, eating well, running)
- Positive feelings
- Absence of negative feelings
- Being normal
- Being involved—having opportunities and experiences
- Achievement
- Independence and choice
- A sense of security
- Good relationships with others (parents, friends, siblings)

A survey of 3000 London children carried out for the Children's Commisioner's Office identified five areas which children perceived as priorities for action to improve health and well-being: violence and safe streets, child abuse, drugs, bullying, and racism.

Measuring or assessing health has not proved easy. There are, however, a number of instruments (questionnaires) which seek to measure health-related quality of life, either for the general population (generic measures) or for those who are suffering from a particular condition or have undergone some intervention or treatment (disease specific measures). These are necessarily subjective, reflecting the perspective of the individual completing them about their own health. The best known examples of generic measures for adults include the SF-36, which measures eight dimensions of health and the EuroQOL, which reduces health to a single dimension. A recent systematic review of measures of child health identified three generic measures for children with sufficiently high scientific validity for use in the general population. These were the CHQ (Child Health Questionnaire), CHIP (Child Health and Illness Profile), and the Warwick Child Health and Morbidity Profile.

What is disease?

Disease represents a deviation from the 'normal' or healthy state. Disease can be considered on many different levels: explanations in terms of cellular and organ dysfunction are the most familiar to doctors, but social scientists and anthropologists have shown that disease can be a social or cultural phenomenon and may be defined differently in different societies.

Disease is a deviation from the 'normal' or healthy state—but it is also a culturally-determined phenomenon.

The cause of illness and disease has been the subject of much philosophical writing over the millennia. In Hippocratic times, the boundaries between medicine, art, religion, and philosophy were less clear than now. Disease was framed in terms of the imbalance of the four humours (blood, phlegm, and black and yellow bile). In Chinese medicine, disease is considered to be caused by an imbalance or lack of harmony between Yin and Yang and between the five elements of earth, fire, water, metal, and wood.

In Western society, the development of germ theory in the nineteenth century led to the concept of 'a single cause for a single disease', which was reinforced by the subsequent success of immunization in preventing disease. However, as non-infectious diseases increased in significance it became evident that this model had serious limitations. It has now been largely replaced with a multifactorial model of causation which is relevant even to infectious diseases, since it is now recognized that the host and the environment play a significant part in their causation, as well as the infective agent. This is explored further below in the discussion of causality and risk.

What is public health?

Definitions of health and disease are clearly of relevance to definitions of public health, but what follows from the above two sections is that the apparently simple questions—'what is health?' and 'what is disease?'—are far from simple to answer. It is not altogether surprising that there have been many different definitions of public health and also of health promotion (see pp. 111–113). The most widely accepted definition of public health is now that of Acheson.

Public health is 'the science and art of promoting health, preventing disease and prolonging life through the organised efforts of society'.

Acheson (1986)

This definition underpins Kohler's definition of child public health presented in the introduction (see p. 2). Public health typically addresses health at the population level rather than at the individual level, and is broadly based and multidisciplinary in its approach.

The Faculty of Public Health has recently identified ten key areas of public health practice which demonstrate the breadth of its scope. They are listed in Table 4.1, with examples to illustrate how each area of practice might relate to child health. Further details of many of the activities listed can be found in later chapters.

Public health had its origins in the nineteenth century and is grounded in the recognition that health is affected by environmental and social conditions, with adverse conditions and lifestyles interacting to create susceptibility to disease. As well as protecting individuals from specific disease-causing agents, public health

Table 4.1 Ten key areas of public health practice

Area of practice	Child health examples
1. Surveillance and assessment of the population's health and well-being	Overseeing the routine child health surveillance system; collecting health data on special groups such as looked-after children or those with disabilities; developing shared databases with other agencies
2. Protecting and promoting health and well-being	Managing communicable disease outbreaks (e.g. meningococcal disease, Hepatitis A) in schools or colleges; overseeing immunization programmes; facilitating local health promotion activities such as 'Five a Day' schemes, 'Safer Ways to School' projects, and cycle safety courses; encouraging the use of smoke alarms
3. Developing quality within an evaluative culture which gets evidence into practice and manages risk	Promoting evidence-based practice in child health for community nurses or GPs; evaluating local services or systems such as inter-agency child protection practice or children's experience in A&E departments
4. Managing, analysing, and interpreting information, knowledge, and statistics	Includes collecting and using national and local data, both routine and ad hoc (e.g. using infant mortality data to monitor UK national inequalities targets; survey of mothers' views of local breast-feeding support services) and undertaking literature reviews to gather, summarize, and disseminate evidence on a particular topic, such as accident prevention
5. Prioritizing and providing professional advice in health and health care	Advising commissioners of health care on priorities for development within child health; input to service planning as a member of local Children's Partnership Group; helping service providers make use of pooled budgets to deliver more effective respite care services for families
6. Policy and strategy development and implementation	Includes both local and national levels e.g membership of Children's Task Force or National Service Framework Implementation Group; developing a local strategy for health care of young asylum seekers or other vulnerable children

Table 4.1 (continued)

Area of practice	Child health examples
7. Developing communities, advocating for health, and reducing inequalities	'Healthy Schools' initiatives; 'SureStart' schemes; involving young people in feedback on health services and service planning; advocating for children's rights; developing peer education schemes on smoking and alcohol or open access health advice services such as 'BodyZones' in schools
8. Strategic leadership for health and well-being across all sectors	Effective co-ordination of multi-agency projects, such as developing innovative child and adolescent mental health services in conjunction with local social services, education departments, and voluntary organizations; making sure children's health and well-being is on the agenda of local government
9. Education, research, and development	Teaching epidemiology and public health principles to health care students and practitioners and others; research on the efficacy of interventions or health services (new vaccines, parenting programmes, preventive dentistry, smoking cessation services for young people)
10. Managing self, people, and resources, and practising ethically	Effective management of 'grass roots' staff such as health visitors and community nurses to maximize the public health benefit of their work; ensuring confidentiality and promoting children's rights

interventions often aim to make general improvements to social and environmental conditions in order to improve the health of the population. The distinction between public health reforms and more general social reforms is not always clear, as improved health may be one of many social goods which are delivered through social reforms such as laws to limit child labour.

Health promotion
The aims of health promotion

Most definitions of health promotion now suggest that its goals are to improve health in the positive, holistic sense enshrined in the WHO definition cited at the beginning of this chapter. They recognize that health depends on the balance of social, mental, and physical well-being and seek to promote all three. Physical well-being is a familiar concept to most of us, but mental and social well-being are perhaps less familiar. Mental well-being has been described by the Mental Health Foundation as positive or good mental health. As the box below makes clear, that encompasses much more than the absence of mental illness:

Good mental health is not just the absence of mental health problems. Individuals with good mental health:

• Develop emotionally, creatively, intellectually, and spiritually

• Initiate, develop, and sustain mutually satisfying relationships

• Face problems, resolve them, and learn from them

• Are confident and assertive

• Are aware of others' needs and empathize with them

• Use and enjoy solitude

• Play and have fun

• Laugh both at themselves and at the world

Mental Health Foundation (2002)

Social well-being reflects the attributes of more than one individual and is thus more complex than physical or mental well-being. It is dependent on the capacity to function as a social being, to form healthy supportive relationships, and to participate positively in community affairs. It is also determined in part by the norms of behaviour in particular societies or communities.

Social well-being depends on the existence of positive social networks to support the individual, and the ability of the individual to contribute positively to those networks. Both the giving and receiving seem to be important. For example, John Helliwell has demonstrated that the *general* level of group membership (e.g. the number of people belonging to social clubs, churches, and religious institutions) in a community contributes to individuals' well-being, even if they do not participate themselves. Conversely, when individuals participate in groups they benefit community well-being as well as their own well-being.

Health promotion seeks to improve physical, mental, and social well-being. At a population level, it aims to improve health for all and to tackle social inequalities in health.

Social capital is a concept which covers many of the components of social well-being and is discussed in more detail below. *Empowerment* is another concept which is important to health promotion because of its impact on social and mental well-being. This term was first used by health promotion practitioners who recognized that agency (the ability to have an influence on the world), self-efficacy (belief in the capacity to have an influence), and personal autonomy (the ability to speak and act independently of others) were vital for health and well-being. Empowerment was the term used to describe the process of enabling people to develop these attributes of well-being. Empowerment is important both at the level of the individual and at the collective level, and health promotion practitioners may aim to empower groups of people or communities to take charge of their own destinies to a greater extent than has been possible in the past.

At a population level, health promotion aims to improve health for all and to tackle social inequalities in health. The WHO's European region has identified two main areas for action on health promotion and disease prevention: firstly, to reduce health inequalities between and within countries, and secondly, to strengthen health as much as to reduce disease. The four principles of 'Health for all in Europe' reflect this agenda:

1. *Ensure equity in health* by reducing the present gap in health status between countries, and between groups within countries.

2. *Add life to years* by ensuring the full development and use of people's integral or residual physical and mental capacity to derive full benefit from and to cope with life in a healthy way.

3. *Add health to life* by reducing disease and disability.

4. *Add years to life* by reducing premature deaths and thereby increasing life expectancy.

Approaches to health promotion

Key examples of the many different definitions of health promotion—some leaning more towards the individual, others towards society—are illustrated in Table 4.2.

The differences of accentuation implicit in these definitions reflect both different belief systems and also change over time. The individual focus derives from the belief that individuals have control over their health-related behaviour and that societal constraints are less important. The 1984 WHO definition encapsulates the idea that individual empowerment is an important 'tool' and is also important in itself for mental and social well-being and therefore health, especially when a lack of empowerment means that a person feels powerless to influence the way they live. Labonte's definition, on the other hand, recognizes that an individual's capacity to change the way in which he or she lives is constrained by the social and physical fabric of society—they may not merely *feel* powerless, but *be* relatively powerless to effect change.

These different definitions have implications for the way health promotion programmes are conceived and implemented. There are generally thought to be at least three levels at which such programmes may operate:

1. the individual level (e.g. health education and individual empowerment)

2. the social or community level (e.g. social action and community empowerment)

3. the policy level (e.g. lobbying and advocacy directed at healthy public policy)

It is usually more effective to combine action at two or three different levels rather than to focus on one. Each is discussed further in the following sections.

Many health promotion activities and programmes include, or are specifically directed at, children and young people: they may seek to promote health and well-being both in the children of the present and for the adults of the future. For example,

Table 4.2 Definitions of health promotion

Lalonde (1974)
A **strategy** 'aimed at informing, influencing and assisting both individuals and organisations so that they will accept more responsibility and be more active in matters affecting mental and physical health'

US Department of Health, Education, and Welfare (1979)
'A **combination** of health education and related organisational, political and economic programs designed to support changes in behavior and in the environment that will improve health'

Green (1980)
'Any combination of health education and related organisational, political and economic **interventions** designed to facilitate behavioural and environmental adaptations that will improve or protect health'

Green and Iverson (1982)
'Any combination of health education and related organisational, economic, and environmental **supports** for behaviour conducive to health'

Perry and Jessor (1983)
'The implementation of **efforts** to foster improved health and well-being in all four domains of health'

Nutbeam (1985)
'The process of enabling people to increase control over the **determinants** of health and thereby improve their health'

WHO (1984, 1986); Epp (1986)
'The **process** of enabling people to increase control over, and to improve, their health'

Goodstadt et al. (1987)
'The maintenance and enhancement of existing levels of health through the implementation of **effective programs, services, and policies**'

Kar (1987)
'The advancement of well-being and the avoidance of health risks by achieving optimal levels of the behavioral, societal, environmental, and biomedical determinants of health'

O'Donnell (1989)
'The **science** and **art** of helping people choose their lifestyles to move toward a state of optimal health'

Labonte and Little (1992)
'Any **activity** or **program** designed to improve social and environmental living conditions such that people's experience of well being is increased'

From Rootman, I. et al. (ed.) (2001). *Evaluation in health promotion. Principles and perspectives*. WHO Regional Publications, European Series, No. 92, p.10. WHO Office for Europe, Copenhagen promoting exercise in young people may both increase their current self-esteem, sporting prowess, and social interactions, and improve their long-term health and life expectancy. A different approach is often needed to ensure that interventions or services are relevant, accessible, and acceptable to the age groups concerned.

Health education

According to Ewles and Simnett, health education

> comprises planned interventions or programmes for people to learn about health, and to undertake voluntary changes in their behaviour.

Knowledge about health and its determinants is important for the maintenance of health; ignorance, on the other hand, is disempowering.

As well as providing information, health education has a role in transferring skills and building self-esteem. Nutbeam describes the outcome of health education in terms of an improvement in *health literacy*—

> cognitive and social skills which determine the motivation and ability of individuals to gain access to, and understand and use information in ways that promote health.

Although it may be delivered at a group, community, or even population level, health education aims to improve the knowledge and skills of individuals, and thus represents the individual end of the health promotion activity spectrum. For example, personal, social and health education (PSHE) in settings such as schools and young offenders institutions has the potential to improve young people's knowledge about the impact of health-related behaviours such as substance misuse or (for a younger age group) road safety.

The relationship between acquisition of knowledge and skills and changes in health-enhancing behaviour is not straightforward, however. Many factors are involved in decision making about, and achievement of, behaviour change and there is wide recognition that didactic teaching is insufficient on its own to alter behaviour. For example, self-awareness and readiness to change are important mediating factors—which are in turn closely related to emotional well-being. Various models have been proposed to elucidate the process and the factors involved in effecting individual behaviour change, thus providing a theoretical framework for effective health promotion programmes. They include the health belief model, the theory of reasoned action, social learning theory, and the stages of change model. Brief outlines are given below.

Health belief model (Rosenstock and Becker) This relies on the concept that individuals hold a number of beliefs about health, including their own susceptibility, the severity of the condition being targeted, and the benefits of and barriers to the recommended preventive actions. All these beliefs influence the individual's likelihood of taking action. Cues to action or strategies to activate might include mass media campaigns, advice from health professionals and others, and experience of the condition in a friend or member of the family. Health promoting activities are framed as influencing the belief systems. You are more likely to act if you think you are likely to get the disease and it is serious, and if you believe that the benefits of taking action outweigh the costs (time, pain, money, inconvenience).

Theory of reasoned action (Azjen and Fishbein) This model holds that your behaviour depends on your intentions, which in turn depend on your attitude (influenced by beliefs about the consequences of the behaviour and the value that you ascribe to these outcomes) and subjective norms (your feelings about other people's perception of the behaviour and how much you care about this). Health promotion interventions are aimed at altering beliefs about the behaviour or perception of the peer group's views. This recognizes that individuals rarely act alone and are influenced by norms set by those around them. Perceived behavioural control makes it easier or harder for a particular individual to act on their intentions based on what power or control each option gives you.

Social learning theory (Rotter) The key concepts are based on an ecological approach: reciprocal determinism (behaviour change results from interaction between the individual and the environment), behavioural capability (knowledge and skills to influence behaviour), expectations (beliefs about likely results of action), and self-efficacy (confidence in ability to take action and persist with it). The main premise is that behavioural change in individuals comes about by change in the social environment.

Stages of change (Prochaska and Di Clemente) This approach is based on understanding that people are at different levels of readiness to take action or change their behaviour at different times in their lives. Health promotion interventions must be appropriate to the stage that the person is at. Five stages are described—precontemplation, contemplation, preparation, action, and maintenance. Health promoting interventions focus on either the thinking stages (e.g. conciousness raising, environmental re-evaluation e.g. non-smoking areas, self re-evaluation) or the doing stages (e.g. facilitating social support, reinforcement management building up personal rewards for desirable actions), and have been found to be more effective if they match the stage the individual has reached in terms of altering their behaviour.

Social capital

Social capital is a relatively new concept in public health and health promotion. The term was coined by social scientists to describe attributes of communities where there is co-operation for mutual benefit, trust in civic institutions, and participation in community affairs. It has been found that people living in such communities experience a number of benefits, including improved health as measured by life expectancy, heart disease, and cancer. As a result, social capital has become an important concept in public health and is coming to be regarded as a determinant of health. We describe it here rather than in Chapter 2 because it is a concept which needs some explanation, because it is important for understanding community approaches to health promotion, and because most of the studies relating social capital to health have been carried out in adults not children. Social capital may therefore be more important for parents than for their children.

> Social capital has become an important concept in public health. It describes attributes of communities where there is co-operation for mutual benefit, trust in civic institutions and participation in community affairs. Social capital can have a positive impact on health—although it is not clear how this happens.

Social cohesion and connectedness are terms which have been included in definitions of social capital. They describe the invisible glue which binds communities of people together, gives them a shared sense of identity, and enables them to work together for the benefit of the whole community. They are generated by social network interaction and can be characterized by feelings of trust and belonging to the community or society, and of interaction and interrelationships. Social capital thus principally reflects attributes of relationships between community members collectively, and to a lesser extent as individuals. There is good evidence from detailed studies in Chicago that the social or organizational characteristics of neighbourhoods explain variations in crime rates that are not attributable to the aggregated demographic characteristics of the individuals within them. In this case it is the 'collective efficacy' (the linkage of mutual trust and willingness to intervene for the common good) of the community in not tolerating crime that acts as a form of informal social control.

Communities with low average income are more likely to have low levels of social capital, but these two determinants of health are independent of one another and it would seem that high social capital may protect members of economically deprived communities from some of the health effects of poverty.

Mechanisms The impact of social capital on health is an example of an epidemiological phenomenon being identified before the mechanisms are clear (see p. 124), and there has been much debate about precisely how social capital affects health. Mechanisms which have been proposed include promotion of the economy through networking and collaborative ventures (economical capital), and the development of skills and competencies (human capital) in the community or group. Social capital may also represent a resource for further development of the community, in that new networks may be built upon older networks using the social relationships, norms and values, trust and information already developed in them. At the simplest level, however, social capital can be seen as a description of supportive, respectful relationships between community members. Such relationships could have a direct effect on health by enhancing emotional well-being and by reducing the stress generated by day-to-day life events. Destructive relationships—those characterized by suspiciousness, exclusion, and fear—could have a direct deleterious effect on health. We have seen in Chapter 2 that there is good evidence that the quality of relationships between parents and their children has an important effect on children's health and, like these relationships, social capital appears to offer a measure of protection from the deleterious effects of poverty. Studies on social capital and adult health may therefore be capturing a similar phenomenon amongst adults.

The box shows one tool which has been developed for measuring social capital.

Measuring social capital

The WHO Health Behaviour of School Children survey in 2001/2002 used a social capital 'package' with four components:

1. Social networks and social support
2. Power and control through engagement
3. Local identity
4. Perception of resources

Although most of the social capital literature focusses on adults, there are some studies relating to children. Coleman found that low social cohesion was the strongest predictor for high school students dropping out of school, and Runyan showed that children from low income areas who scored high on a social capital index performed consistently better on developmental and behavioural testing than their peers. An ecological model proposed by Earls and Carlson ties family relationships and community relationships together, envisioning family processes and individual development as embedded in community and other macrosocial structures.

This might be considered a somewhat reductionist model of child well-being. It implies that all that society—and families—need to do to promote children's well-being is to supervise and control them and that self-efficacy is the only aspect of mental health that matters. Earls derived the model from work in the context of a violent or disruptive neighbourhood, but warmth and affection, positive regard, and approval within the family are also important for emotional well-being, along with the traditional 'limit setting', supervisory parental role.

Despite criticisms of the literature on social capital, there is no doubt that it is an important concept for health promotion and may modify the impact of poverty on health.

There has been criticism of the term 'social capital' on the grounds that it is perceived to have a poor theoretical framework and that it simplifies a range of social phenomena to 'one true measure' which can be substituted for the social understanding required for humane social policy and public health practice. Others have suggested that the concept is just not applicable to children, especially as in some

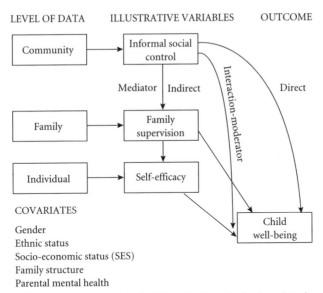

LEVEL OF DATA   ILLUSTRATIVE VARIABLES   OUTCOME

Fig. 4.1 Multilevel analytical model of child well-being. (Earls, F. and Carlson, M. (2001). The social ecology of child health and well-being. With permission, from the Annual Review of Public Health, Volume **22**:143–66. ©2001 by Annual Reviews www.annualreviews.org

guises social capital emphasises civicness, institutions, and public affairs, and these are social activities from which children are often excluded.

In spite of these criticisms and a lack of precise understanding of the mechanisms involved, the phenomena described in the social capital literature are undoubtedly of importance to health promotion. In the context of social inequalities, health promotion practitioners need to address the question: is it most effective to foster social capital and social cohesion in disadvantaged communities with poor levels of 'connectedness', or should interventions be aimed at improving income equality? This is an important question for everyone concerned with tackling health inequalities and improving the lot of the worst off in society. Most of those working with disadvantaged communities would consider that both approaches are important—that interventions should be directed both at income improvement and at developing local networks and facilities, trust, and support. The latter approach depends on harnessing the close co-operation and involvement of members of the community, through activities such as community participation or community development.

Community approaches to health promotion

Community participation Community participation is the process of working with a community to improve its social capital, usually with the aim of improving the health and well-being of the community and its members. Much of the experience of community participation comes from developing countries, but it has also been used in disadvantaged communities in the UK and other developed countries since the nineteenth century. Rifkin suggests four reasons why community participation in health is desirable:

1. Interventions to change behaviour and lifestyle—and thereby to improve health—can only succeed through individuals' conscious participation.
2. Participation of users in the planning and running of services should improve the appropriateness of those services for the population.
3. Communities have untapped resources which may be directed towards promoting health concerns, through the involvement of community members in the financing, building, and running of health facilities.
4. It is the right and duty of people to participate in activities affecting their daily lives.

Community development Community development is a means of assisting community participation, especially in fragmented communities with high social needs, through the use of skilled workers from outside the community who work alongside members of the local community on topics identified by the community. These might include developing after school activities or youth groups, a 'Safer Ways to School' scheme, or a parent and toddler group.

It is important that the views of children and young people are taken into account as well as those of their parents. The role of the worker is to assist the organizational process while remaining in the background him or herself, aiming to empower community members and enable them to develop the skills and attitudes necessary to bring about change. 'Healthy Schools' schemes reflect the principles of community development, with children and young people being offered the chance to take control of and improve aspects of school life, addressing what they perceive to be important problems, sometimes through participation in a school council. Proposed action might include starting a breakfast club or sports activities at lunchtime, altering the layout of the playground or the management of break times to tackle bullying, running a healthy snacks stall, or raising funds for new play equipment.

Community diagnosis The term community diagnosis is used for the process of assessing health needs within a community, which may involve community participation techniques. To make a community diagnosis is to identify the problems, needs, and resources of a community in order to develop appropriate solutions to these problems. Community diagnosis should include both priorities identified by professionals via epidemiological methods, and locally determined (psychosociological) priorities. These are not necessarily the same. For example, professionals might identify smoking, alcohol abuse, and poor diet as the basis for a community's health problems, while local families might identify poor housing, safety concerns, lack of play space or child care, and inadequate local shops as the main health issues for them. (See Chapter 6 for a fuller discussion.)

Advocacy

According to the *Oxford Dictionary*, to be an advocate is 'to plead or raise one's voice in favour of [a cause or person]; to defend or recommend publicly'. In other words, advocacy is 'to stand beside', not 'to do for'. In public health terms, advocacy and lobbying ('seeking to influence legislators') are often activities directed at the third level of health promotion, which seeks to encourage healthy public policy—that is, policies which favour health rather than putting obstacles in the way of it. Examples of healthy public policy might include the provision of cycle paths and safe routes to school at a local level, and the banning of tobacco advertising at national level. Public health professionals have an important role to play in raising health policy issues and putting pressure on governments and others to make changes in policy.

But advocacy can operate at an individual level as well as a population level. At the individual level, advocacy means making a commitment to support the child and family beyond the immediate issues related to their medical condition. It is integral to the work of many professionals involved with children—paediatricians, social workers, community nurses, GPs—because of a shared wish to meet all of a child's health-related and social needs within the context of his or her family and community. Factors outside the realm of direct health care provision (including family, educational, social, cultural, spiritual, economic, environmental, and political factors) often inhibit children's ability to achieve their full potential—particularly among children from disadvantaged families.

> Advocacy can operate at the individual level, supporting and arguing the case for a child or family, or at the population level, to promote healthy public policy.

Child health advocacy often begins in this way, with an individual patient, and may extend into local, regional, or national work in a public health capacity, sometimes following through the same issues on a more general level—perhaps lobbying for certain services to be provided for the local population, rather than just for a particular child or children, or opposing cuts in service which will affect both known and unknown children.

Examples of opportunities for advocacy on an *individual* level include supporting an application for rehousing for a child with chronic serous otitis media and recurrent respiratory infections who lives in an overcrowded, damp house; writing to the school about the emotional consequences for a child with a disability who is in a mainstream school but falling behind, being bullied, and receiving inadequate teaching support; or helping teachers to feel more confident in dealing with a child with asthma in the classroom when they are reluctant to provide medication within the school setting.

Examples of opportunities for advocacy affecting a specific *population* include supporting a school campaign to improve safety in the streets nearby, promoting the emotional and social needs of local teenagers by lobbying local government for better youth facilities in the locality, or lobbying government to change outdated legislation which allows parents to use corporal punishment on their children.

Effective advocacy has a number of important elements and requires particular skills which those trained to deliver services (health, social care, education, etc.) may or may not possess, but can certainly learn and practice. The boxes below set out what advocacy involves and what skills professionals need in order to be effective advocates.

Essential components of advocacy for child health

- A problem within the system which is obstructing children's care, or a policy issue which is adverse to children's health
- The potential for individual or group intervention (such as lobbying) to bring about change
- Will and determination to make things better and to improve the system for children
- Presenting a good, succinct case and being prepared to see it through

Skills needed for advocacy

- Understanding of political system
- Lack of political bias
- Ability to manage change
- Assertiveness
- Media skills
- Holistic approach to health and health care
- Good team working and networking
- Ability to prioritize
- Persistence, patience, and tolerance of long time-scales

Epidemiological concepts: causality and risk

Our ability to intervene and to effect changes in the health of a population relies on an understanding of the factors involved in triggering ill health or promoting positive health. Causality and risk are key concepts here, and they are worth exploring in some detail.

Causality

Causality can be defined as 'the operation or relation of cause and effect'. As we have already seen, there is rarely a single cause–effect relationship in triggering disease. Why is it, for example, that one child in a nursery appears to catch every infection which he or she encounters, while others escape many of them despite having the same exposure to infectious agents?

Rothman defines a cause of a specific disease event as an

antecedent event, condition, or characteristic that was necessary for the occurrence of the disease at the moment that it occurred.

Recognizing the interaction of several different factors, he uses the term 'sufficient cause' to describe a complete causal mechanism or a set of minimal conditions and events that are necessary in order to produce disease.

> There is rarely a single cause–effect relationship in triggering disease usually several factors are involved. It is easier to demonstrate *association* with a disease then causality.

It is often easier, however, to show which factors are *associated* with a disease or illness than to say which *cause* it. Bradford Hill proposed a set of criteria which can help us distinguish the two and determine whether the relationship between exposure to a particular factor and developing a particular disease is a causal or coincidental association. These criteria are set out in Table 4.3.

Table 4.3 Bradford Hill criteria for causation

Criteria	Comments
Strength—the ratio of incidence to exposure, or the relative risk (see below) (e.g. passive smoking and childhood asthma).	The stronger the association is, the less likely it is to be due to some other coincidental factor (a 'confounder').
Consistency—the repeated observation of an association in different populations (e.g. vitamin D deficiency and rickets).	This again makes it unlikely that the association is due to another factor, which might well vary between different populations.
Specificity—a particular cause leads to the same particular event in all cases (e.g. congenital limb malformations seen in babies exposed to thalidomide in *utero*).	This criterion has been criticized on the grounds that single exposures may lead to many effects (e.g. smoking leads to a myriad of diseases as well as being a 'cause' of lung cancer).
Temporality—the cause precedes the effect (e.g. an inflamed arm following immunization).	Logically, effect must follow cause.
Biological gradient—a dose-response relationship, where higher levels of exposure lead to greater risk or more serious disease (e.g. lower iron intake leads to more severe anaemia).	There are two criticisms of this criterion: (a) some relationships are *threshold* effects as opposed to gradients (e.g. the association of diethylstilboestrol in pregnancy and vaginal cancer in the offspring) (b) A confounding factor may also have a dose–response relationship: e.g. the non-causal association between birth order and risk of Down's syndrome, which is really due to maternal age.

Table 4.3 (continued)

Criteria	Comments
Coherence—the proposed cause–effect relationship does not conflict with what is already known of the natural history and biology of the disease.	This is a similar concept to plausibility. The presence of conflicting information may be useful in refuting a hypothetical causal link, but this information may itself be mistaken or misinterpreted, so care is needed here.
Experimental evidence—evidence from laboratory experiments on animals or intervention studies in humans shows that removing the exposure reduces the incidence of the disease.	This is a *test* of causality as opposed to a criterion for establishing it, and in many instances evidence of this kind is unavailable.
Analogy—a similar causal relationship is already well-established (e.g. smoking is known to cause lung cancer, which strengthens the case for a causal association with other kinds of cancer).	As for plausibility, the absence of analogies only reflects a lack of imagination or experience, not the falsity of the hypothesis.
Plausibility—the existence of a biological explanation for the association (e.g. effects on specific organs at cellular level or on cell division).	This depends on possible mechanisms having been identified and tested, which is not always the case even for relationships which do turn out to be causal—but it is still a useful criterion.

Source: Adapted from the Oxford textbook of Public Health (1997); **12**:626–7

One key point is that it is not always necessary to understand the *mechanisms* involved in a causal relationship in order to be sure it exists and to act on it. Famous examples of important public health interventions in which the mechanism behind a causal association was (or is) incompletely understood include the removal of the handle from the Broad Street pump to halt the spread of cholera in Victorian London, the recommendation to stop smoking in order to reduce the risk of lung cancer, the 'Back to Sleep' campaign in the prevention of sudden infant death syndrome. These examples arguably illustrate separate phases of our understanding of causality and its link with preventive action which Susser has described as different 'eras' in the evolution of epidemiology. We are now entering the era of eco-epidemiology which takes advantage of combining emerging biomedical technologies (genetic, imaging, etc.) and information technology (see Table 4.4).

It is worth noting that causality can be considered both in epidemiological and in socio-anthropological terms. The epidemiological approach consists of the scientific study of patterns of disease and of cause and effect, as outlined above, whereas the socio-anthropological perspective reflects the beliefs and understanding of parents and children about the causes of disease and ill health. An extension of the eco-epidemiological methodology is to include the privileged epistemological perspective of community members in the definition of variables, the design of measurements

Table 4.4 Different eras in the evolution of epidemiology

Era	Paradigm	Analytic approach	Preventive approach
Sanitary statistics (first half of 19th century)	Miasma: poisoning by foul emanations from soil, air, and water	Demonstrate clustering of morbidity and mortality	Introduce drainage, sewage, sanitation
Infectious disease (late 19th century through first half of 20th century)	Germ theory: single agents relate one to one to specific diseases	Laboratory isolation and culture from disease sites, experimental transmission and reproduction of lesions	Interrupt transmission (vaccines, isolation of the affected through quarantine and fever hospitals and ultimately antibiotics)
Chronic diseases epidemiology (latter half of the 20th century)	Black box: exposure related to outcome, without necessity for intervening factors or pathogenesis	Risk ratio of exposure to outcome at individual level in populations	Control risk factors by modifying lifestyle (diet, exercise, etc.), agent (guns, food, etc.), or environment (pollution, passive smoking, etc.)
Eco-epidemiology (emerging)	Chinese boxes: relations within and between localized structures organized in a hierarchy of levels	Analysis of determinants and outcomes at different levels of organization: within and across contexts (using new information systems) and in depth (using biomedical techniques)	Apply both information and biomedical technology to find leverage at efficacious levels from contextual to new molecular

Source: Susser, M. and Susser, E. Choosing a future for epidemiology: II. From black box to chinese boxes and eco-epidemiology. *American Journal of Public Health Medicine*; **86**:5, 674–7, permission sought.

and interventions, the data collection, and the analysis. This aims to ensure that research design reflects the way people in the study population experience life. The child public health professional and researcher alike will find a rich source of emerging data with respect to service redesign based on these interelated perspectives.

Causality can be considered both in epidemiological and in socio-anthropological terms—the latter reflecting the beliefs and understanding of parents and children about the causes of disease and ill health.

Risk

Risk can be defined as 'a chance or possibility of danger, loss, injury, or other adverse consequences'. In health terms, a risk factor is one which exposes an individual or population to the chance or possibility of disease or ill health. Risk factors may be factors in the environment, or chemical, psychological, physiological, or genetic elements which predispose an individual to the development of a disease.

The nature, measurement, and communication of risk is a complex area in public health. Exposure to a risk factor does not necessarily lead to the development of the disease it 'causes', nor can we explain why some exposed people develop the disease and others do not, because we do not usually know precisely which factors are involved and how these different factors interact. For the unlucky toddler already described, who catches every infection 'going round' the nursery, there must be other factors apart from exposure to viruses which increase his or her risk of succumbing to infection. Although we are uncertain exactly what these factors are, they might include his or her home environment, the adequacy of nursery staff handwashing, emotional stress, whether the parents smoke, sleep patterns, exercise, environmental temperature and humidity, and nutritional factors.

> Risk factors predispose individuals to disease, but do not necessarily lead to the development of the disease. Often the best we can do is to work out the average risk for a group of people with the same level of exposure to a particular factor.

What we can do, however, is to work out the average risk posed to people exposed to a certain hazard or agent by looking at the incidence of disease in all those exposed and comparing it with the incidence in those not exposed (see further discussion of statistical descriptors below). For hazards which are not 'all or nothing' (e.g. factors such as poor nutrition or lack of exercise, rather than exposure to the rubella virus), a graded approach may be used, categorizing people according to their level of exposure and the level of risk this carries. Risks assessed in this way can be described as 'indicators' in predicting ill health among certain groups.

In essence, therefore, this approach involves assigning the same average risk to every member of a particular group or population. It has important shortcomings, one of which is the so-called 'ecological fallacy', which applies to any situation where people are considered in groups and conclusions are drawn about the group as a whole without examining the individuals. The argument goes that the features of the individuals who are affected by the condition in question may differ from those of others in the group. The group's 'defining characteristic' (the reason we have grouped them together—e.g. the risk factor we are looking at) may not after all be the key causal factor.

For example, suppose there is a high incidence of congenital abnormalities in babies born in a town near a chemical plant where many of the local population are employed. Comparing the incidence of abnormalities in this town with those in other local towns, and relating them to the proportion of parents employed in the chemical factory, a local investigator concludes that there is good evidence to suggest that the chemical factory is the cause of the abnormalities, and the population of factory workers is identified as at increased risk of having babies with congenital abnormalities. However, when the actual cases are examined, it turns out that very few of their parents work at the factory, and a totally different explanation presents itself—perhaps they are members of the same extended family and share a genetic mutation. In this example, it would be relatively simple to study the individuals concerned and expose the ecological fallacy, but where larger populations or more common conditions are involved—or where the 'risk' is harder to define individually or consists not of black and white but shades of grey—then it can be much harder to detect the flaw in the supposed cause–effect relationship.

The explosion of genetic phenotyping may allow us to assign more precise risk estimates to individuals as some of the 'hidden' factors involved in mediating cause and effect relationships may turn out to be genetic and measurable. For now, however, group effects are often the best we can do, and much of the science of epidemiology relies upon them. They have been good enough to determine much of what we know about the determinants of public health today.

Statistical descriptors of risk

Various different terms and concepts can be useful in describing and quantifying risk.

Absolute risk This is the incidence of a condition in a certain population. It is usually expressed as a decimal or a percentage e.g. 2% or 0.02. The absolute risk of a condition may vary between different populations e.g. those living in different countries or areas, or those who are or are not exposed to a risk factor.

Relative risk This is the ratio of the incidence of a condition in an exposed population to its incidence in an unexposed population. The 'strength' of association described in Table 4.4 above is greater when this figure is higher. For example, if 20% of children whose diets contain less than the recommended daily allowance of vitamin A develop nightblindness, compared to 0.1% of children taking the recommended levels, then the relative risk associated with inadequate intake would be 20 ÷ 0.1, or 200. Because it is a ratio, relative risk does not have units.

Another name for relative risk is the **risk ratio**. The **odds ratio** and **rate ratio** are similar concepts, measured in slightly different ways, which can be used as an approximation of the relative risk. Risk, odds, and rate use the same *numerator* (the number of new cases seen in a population in a given time), but different *denominators*. For risk, the denominator is the size of the population (strictly speaking, the number of disease-free people at the start). For odds, it is the number of people who do NOT become cases within the given time. For rate, it is the total person time at risk (i.e. the number of disease-free people multiplied by the time period).

It is often important to know both the absolute and the relative risk in order to make a meaningful assessment of risk. For example, suppose the relative risk for those exposed to a particular hazard was 20. If the absolute risk in the general (unexposed) population was 2%, this would give the exposed group a 40% (20×2) chance of developing the disease or condition. If, however, the absolute risk in the unexposed population was 0.002%, or 2 per hundred thousand, then the exposed group's chance of developing the disease would only be 0.04%, or 40 per hundred thousand—a much less worrying statistic.

Attributable risk This is the amount of risk in an **exposed** population which can be attributed to their exposure to the risk factor concerned. For example, suppose the risk of Brown's disease in a population of children exposed to a certain environmental agent is 20%, and the risk in the unexposed population is 2%. We can say that of the 20 cases per hundred children seen in the exposed population, 2 would be expected anyway because of the background risk in the general population, and an additional 18 occur as a result of being exposed. The attributable risk is therefore 18%. It can be calculated as the risk in the exposed group (R_e) minus the risk in the unexposed group (R_o): here, 20%–2% = 18%.

Sometimes attributable risk is expressed as a proportion of the overall risk in the exposed population—in this example, $18 \div 20 = 0.9$, or 90%. This is called the attributable risk percentage or *aetiologic fraction*—the proportion of the exposed population's risk which is due to their exposure. It can be calculated as $(R_e - R_o) \div R_e$.

As the baseline incidence of a condition in the general (unexposed) population goes up, the aetiologic fraction goes down, because a higher proportion of cases in the exposed population are attributable to their background risk rather than to exposure to the risk factor. In the example above, if the risk of Brown's disease in the unexposed population was 12% and the risk in the population exposed to the hazard was 30%, the attributable risk would still be 18% but the aetiologic fraction would be $18 \div 30 = 0.6$, or 60%.

Population attributable risk This is the amount of risk in the **total** population which is attributable to the exposure. It reflects the attributable risk in the exposed population and the proportion of the total population who are exposed. Using the Brown's disease example again, let us suppose that 10% of the population are exposed to the environmental risk factor. Using the initial figures of 2% risk in the unexposed population and 20% risk in the exposed population, we can examine the overall incidence of Brown's disease in a hypothetical representative sample of, say, 1000 people. Of these, 900 will be unexposed, and 2% of 900 = 18 of them will develop the disease. The remaining 100 will be exposed, and 20% of 100 = 20 of them will develop the disease. The total risk in the population is therefore $18 + 20 = 38$ cases in 1000 people (or 3.8%), of which we know 18 are due to exposure to the risk factor (the attributable risk calculated above). The *population* attributable risk is therefore 18 cases per 1000 people, or 1.8%.

Again, rather than working out from first principles each time, there are mathematical formulae for calculating the population attributable risk. It can be calculated *either* as the risk in the population as a whole (R_t) minus the risk in the unexposed population (R_o) *or* as the attributable risk multiplied by the proportion of the population exposed. Here, the first calculation would give us 3.8%–2% = 1.8%, and the second method would give us 18% $\times$ 0.1 (which is also 1.8%).

Number needed to harm This is a related concept. It is the number of people who would need to be exposed to a risk factor in order for one additional person to be harmed or to develop the condition concerned. In the example above, we know that exposing 100 people to the risk factor results in 18 additional cases of Brown's disease. The number of people who would need to be exposed to result in one additional case is therefore 100 ÷ 18 = 5.5. This is the number needed to harm.

Perception of risk

As well as measuring and evaluating risk using the methods described above, public health practitioners also have an important role in communicating risk to the population and helping them to understand and to respond to it—for example, by changing their behaviour (e.g. altering their babies' sleeping position to reduce the risk of SIDS) or by lobbying for action by others (e.g. adding fluoride to drinking water to reduce the incidence of dental caries in local children). The perception of risk by the public may not always be as professionals expect, however. Hazards over which people have no control (such as landfill sites or nuclear installations) may be perceived as more threatening, as may new or unfamiliar threats (such as BSE). Although far more children are killed by a parent or carer than by a stranger—and very many more by cars than by any human being—the publicity and distress which follows a child murder by an unknown assailant reflects and feeds intense public fear of such events.

> Public health practitioners have an important role in communicating risk to the public and helping them to understand and to respond to it.

Children's perceptions of risk may be influenced by the views of their parents, teachers, or others, but may also differ significantly from them. Risks which children can visualize (again, the dangerous stranger) are often more worrying, and they tend to perceive living things (e.g. people or dogs) as more threatening than inanimate objects such as cars. However, unseen dangers ('germs', poisons, or aliens under the bed) can also capture the imagination and be perceived as a serious risk. Children may also connect events to generate their own causal theories in a way adults may not expect: 'grandpa died in hospital, so if I have to go there I'll die too'.

Communicating risk

One important challenge is how best to communicate the risk of disease or an intervention. Risk communication can be defined as the open two-way exchange of information and opinion about risk, leading to a better understanding and better decisions being made. This definition acknowledges the two-way nature of the process as opposed to the unidirectional doctor to patient route. The context of risk is important. Risks may be voluntary or imposed; they may be familiar or unknown (which may affect the degree of dread); and they may be concentrated or dispersed over time. An example which neonatal intensive care specialists and parents regularly face is how best to weigh up the intensity of resuscitative and maintenance measures for an extremely premature infant and the risks of later serious handicap. This dilemma is of course extended to the population level when rationing decisions have to be made about health care services. One of the most common dilemmas facing GPs is communicating the risks of a certain intervention, for example, the benefits of antibiotics for acute otitis media in children against possible harm or no effect. The use of diagrams can be very helpful in communicating such ideas (see Fig. 4.2).

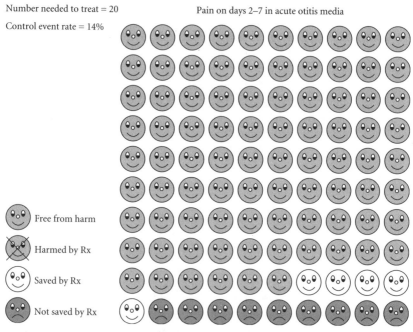

Fig. 4.2 Portrayal of risks and benefits of treatment with antibiotics for otitis media designed with Rx, a program that calculates numbers needed to treat from the pooled results of a meta-analysis and produces a graphical display of the result. (Source: Edwards, A., Elwyn, G., and Mulley, A. *BMJ* (2002) **324**:827–30, with permission from the BMJ Publishing Group.)

Some other evidence-based approaches in communicating risk are shown in the box:

◆ Avoid using areas or volumes to depict quantities.

◆ Absolute risks (with appropriate scales) should be given greater prominence than relative risks—in both information for patients and journals for professionals.

◆ Comparison with everyday tasks is valuable, such as where the risk can be compared with other well-known risks (car accident).

◆ The influence of 'framing' of risk should be countered by using dual representations (loss and gain, mortality and survival).

Risk and positive concepts of health

As difficult as it is to identify accurately all the risk factors for a given disease, it is even more challenging to describe the risk factors pertaining to maintenance of good health. Graham has attempted this by describing the minimum conditions for good health: shelter, food, and social cohesion. In other words, there are certain preconditions for maintenance of a baseline of general positive health. However, there have been no attempts to attach numerical values to the risks of good health associated with, for example, lack of shelter.

One of the problems with the application of the risk model to the promotion of health, as opposed to the prevention of disease, is that, because it has been developed with disease prevention in mind, risks are determined with respect to individual diseases. So, for example, we can describe the level of risk of lung cancer for people who smoke compared to those who do not. We can even describe the different levels of risk of lung cancer according to the number of cigarettes smoked per day. However, smoking is a risk factor, not just for lung cancer, but also for a host of other diseases including other cancers, heart disease, and even osteoporosis. Smoking therefore creates susceptibility to a wide range of diseases—and can be said to create **general susceptibility** to ill health. Emotional distress or stress appears to work in the same way, interfering with a number of bodily mechanisms and creating susceptibility to a wide range of illnesses from infections to hypertension and from coronary artery disease to musculoskeletal disease.

In the field of international child health, we have seen that malnutrition is associated with a huge range of diseases. The idea that a single agent or factor can cause many health problems, like the idea that most diseases have a range of different causes, runs counter to the belief that there is a single cause for a single disease, which has been prevalent in medical thinking since the development of the germ theory of disease in the nineteenth century.

Some risk factors—such as smoking or malnutrition—do not just predispose to one disease but create general susceptibility to a range of conditions.

It is clear from the discussion above that certain groups or populations of individuals may be at different risk of disease from others. This is explored further in the next section.

Populations

Populations are useful in establishing *denominators*, which are essential in order to calculate rates or risks of certain conditions (see above). We can find out from the cancer registry how many cases there are of childhood leukaemia in a local population, but in order to compare this incidence with that in other areas, we need to know the size of the population in which the cases occurred.

There are many types of population to which children belong, and which might be useful as denominators. Examples include:

♦ *geographical* or spatially defined populations—a borough or locality, or a health visitor's 'patch'

♦ *administrative* populations—such as a GP caseload, a school, or a primary care organization population

♦ *at risk* populations e.g. those on the child protection register, unimmunized children, or those from traveller families

♦ *target populations* for screening or preventive programmes

Children can also be divided into *age groups* e.g. neonatal, infant, preschool, school-age, adolescent. These populations are clearly not mutually exclusive.

> Populations are used to establish denominators, which are needed to calculate rates or risks of disease. Examples include geographical populations, practitioner caseloads, schools, and age groups.

The focus of a child health professional's interest, or of a specific intervention, might be aimed at several overlapping categories.

Geographical populations

It is possible to relate health data to population data within different geographical areas in order to assess the health of a given small-area population and make comparisons between different areas. This can be done at a number of levels:

Enumerator districts are the areas within which a single census enumerator is responsible for distributing and collecting census forms.

Local authority 'wards' are commonly used: census data can be converted automatically to this unit, which has more meaning for individuals and service planners. Ward data can then be aggregated into larger areas, such as local authority districts—but only where the boundaries of the larger area correspond to those of the wards. This can cause difficulty if, say, a primary care organization's population is required, and its boundaries cut across ward boundaries.

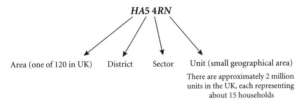

Fig. 4.3 'Anatomy' of a postcode.

Postcodes are increasingly being used as a means of defining and counting populations. Because they represent smaller areas than wards or enumerator districts, they offer greater flexibility in 'reconstituting' larger populations (such as those within PCTs or other primary care organizations). If all the postcodes within a particular population area are known, then the size and composition of that population can be calculated (Fig. 4.3).

Other kinds of population

It is often useful to be able to divide children into different populations or categories in order to analyse the different level of risk experienced by each group. This helps us to understand the role and significance of risk factors in child health, and ultimately to devise interventions designed to promote the health of children. The examples below illustrate this.

Categorization by birth weight

Birth registration is a key source of information about the number of children in an area. It was first established as a statutory duty in the UK in 1874, and parents are still required to register the infant's name and other details within six weeks of delivery. Hospitals also supply data about each birth, which is combined with the registration data by the Office of National Statistics (ONS). One way in which this information is used is to categorize births into different weight bands:

- Low birth weight (LBW) <2500 g
- Very low birth weight (VLBW) <1500 g
- Extremely low birth weight (ELBW) <1000 g

The risk of certain conditions such as cerebral palsy (CP) among babies in different groups can then be compared (see Table 1.4, p.21). Table 1.4 clearly shows the increasing risk of CP with lower birth weight. Using the concepts described above, low birth weight is a risk factor for CP, and the relative risk of CP increases with each decrease in birth weight. This sort of data is invaluable when planning services for high-risk groups of children leaving the neonatal intensive care unit. There has been a two-fold increase in the low birth weight-specific rates of CP in the last 30 years, reflecting considerable improvements in survival at the expense of increased rates of disability. The data is also useful in promoting preventive measures designed to reduce the incidence of low birth weight, such as good antenatal care and maternal nutrition.

Categorization by social class

Since the 1921 Census, the UK has used a system of five (or six) social class categories based on the occupation of the 'head of household'. The rankings were intended to reflect wealth and culture, the latter being equated with a 'combination of knowledge and skill which enables a person to use his purchasing power wisely' (T.H.C. Stevenson, Statistical Superintendent of the General Registrar's Office). For children, social class is obviously ascribed in terms of their parents' (almost always father's) occupation. The categories are illustrated in Table 4.5.

These categories were initially used to describe the large differences in infant mortality rates between different strata in society. Even today, there are still major differences in mortality, morbidity, and behaviour patterns in both children and parents belonging to different social classes, as we saw in Chapter 2.

A further example concerns consulting ratios in general practice, which are higher among children living in council housing than those living in owner-occupied housing for most major causes of consultation. The differences are largest for conditions classed as serious, where consulting ratios among children in council housing are 20% higher than those in owner-occupied housing. Consulting ratios for diseases of the nervous system, however, show a reversed social class trend, with higher consultation rates among higher social classes.

Inequalities in health have continued to increase in the UK although it has become more prosperous and the general level of health has improved, and Children in lower social classes can be seen as an at-risk population for many conditions and causes of ill health. Data on differentials between social classes is crucial in driving the important public health agenda aimed at reducing inequalities in health, and in monitoring the impact of interventions designed to improve the health of the worst off.

However, the traditional social class classification system has important disadvantages: it is based on the occupation of the head of household (normally male)—thus children whose parents have never worked do not have a social class, and women whose partners are unemployed or have a job which belongs to a lower category than their own may be inappropriately classified. There may also be wide variations of income within one social class. A new system, the National Statistics Socio-economic Classification, is being introduced in the UK to replace social class classification, and should overcome some of these problems. Further approaches to assessing social inequalities are discussed below.

Table 4.5 Social class categorization

Social class I	Professionals e.g. doctors and lawyers
Social class II	Intermediate e.g. teachers, nurses, managers
Social class IIIN	Skilled non manual e.g. clerks
Social class IIIM	Skilled manual e.g. coalminers, technicians, ambulance drivers
Social class IV	Partly skilled manual e.g. postmen, bus conductors
Social class V	Unskilled manual e.g. porters, ticket collectors, general labourers

Source: ONS

Measuring poverty and social disadvantage

We have seen that poverty and social disadvantage are important risk factors or determinants of health. It is therefore important to be able to quantify them, in order to examine the relationship and assess the health risk to different populations which results. There is no generally accepted single method of measuring poverty, but a number of different approaches are useful in quantifying poverty and income inequality.

> There are many ways of measuring poverty and income inequality—subjective consensus measures, indices based on local health and social data, and comparative measures are all used to examine the extent of poverty in different areas or countries.

The Gini coefficient

This is a way of comparing income inequality in different countries. It is derived from a Lorenz curve, which is a graph plotting (a) the cumulative income distribution in a particular country, divided into population groups ranked from smallest to largest share of the national income, and (b) a straight diagonal line which represents a hypothetical cumulative distribution where incomes are identical throughout society (see Fig. 4.4). The further the 'actual' curve sags away from the 'hypothetical' straight line, the greater the inequality of income distribution. The Gini coefficient is derived by comparing the area between the two lines with the total area under the straight line, obtaining a value between 0 and 1. The nearer the figure is to one, the more unequal the income distribution within the country.

Consensus or 'subjective' poverty measures

These are based on the opinions of representative samples of the population. They list the basic necessities of life and the proportion of the population who cannot

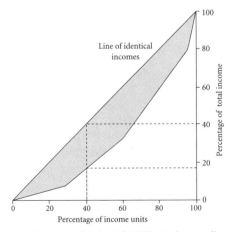

Fig. 4.4 The Lorenz curve. Source: Alcock, P. (1993). Understanding Poverty, Macmillan.

Table 4.6 MORI/London Weekend Television index of deprivation, 1983

Item	% describing as necessary	% lacking item	% lacking because can't afford
3 meals/day for children	82	7	4
2 pairs all-weather shoes	78	15	11
Toys for children	71	5	3
Holiday away from home	63	30	23
Children's leisure equipment	57	17	13

afford them—or calculate the cost of purchasing these necessities, enabling assessment of how far certain income levels fall short of this minimum requirement.

In one study, 18 adult necessities and 18 child necessities were listed; extreme poverty was defined as those adults or children without access to seven or more items because of lack of resources. Table 4.6 shows a sample of the items.

Townsend invited the opinions of a representative sample of adult Londoners in 1986 on the level of disposable income that they regarded as adequate for life and work. The finding was that the levels of income judged to be needed for different family types were on average 60% higher than the means-tested state benefits for which such family types would be eligible.

Geographical measures

These are commonly used in the UK to define and describe the extent of poverty and deprivation within certain areas (such as electoral wards) using information from the census. The Jarman Index uses an eight-item score:

1. % of elderly living alone
2. % of population under five years
3. % of one-parent families
4. % in social class 5
5. % unemployed
6. % living in overcrowded accommodation
7. % changing address in past year
8. % ethnic minority population

This index is widely used in general practice but has the disadvantage of combining demographic indicators with measures of deprivation. The Townsend Index uses only deprivation indicators:

1. % of unemployed
2. % of households which are overcrowded

3. % of households lacking a car

4. % of households not owning their house

The figures below illustrate mapping using the Townsend Deprivation scores.
The most recent example is the UK government's Department of Transport,
London and the Regions (DTLR) Index of Multiple Deprivation 2000, which is more
comprehensive and up to date than either Jarman or Townsend, and is available by

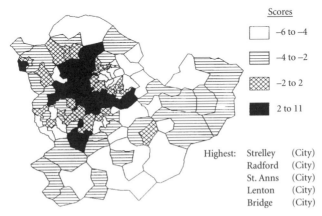

Fig. 4.5 Townsend deprivation scores by electoral ward for Nottingham Health District.
(Source: York Economic Consortium.)

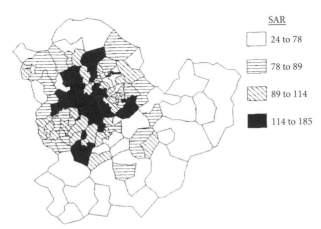

Fig. 4.6 Standardized admission ratios (SARs) for accidents, all ages, in Nottingham
Health District.

ward, with all 8000 or so wards in the country ranked by their overall deprivation score. It includes data from a range of different sources and covers six domains:

Access

—to a post office, food shop, GP, and primary school

Education

—including qualifications among adults and school attendance / college enrolment among children and young people

Employment

—including unemployment claimants and those accessing incapacity and disablement allowance

Health

—including mortality ratios for men and women, limiting longstanding illness, and infant mortality

Housing

—including homelessness and overcrowding

Income

—including income support and family credit recipients

The EU definition of comparative poverty

This commonly used measure compares the extent of poverty in different countries or areas. It is based on households with incomes less than 50% of the national average. Figs. 1.10 and 1.11 in Chapter 1 show the proportion of the total and child population in the UK with incomes below this level, and the changes which have occurred over the last decade or so.

Disease prevention

Disease prevention is related to health promotion, but is a more specifically medical endeavour. As its name suggests, it is concerned primarily with preventing specific

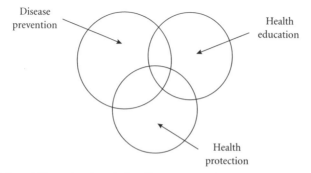

Fig. 4.7 Tannahill overlapping circles. (Source: Downie, R.S., Tannahill, C., Tannahill, A. (1996). *Health Promotion: Models and Values*. Oxford University Press, Oxford.)

diseases. It includes, for example, not only immunization programmes and infection control policies, but also a wide range of other activities, and encompasses measures such as risk factor reduction which often have a more general benefit for health. A useful diagram produced by Tannahill describes the close interrelationship between prevention, health education, and health protection, seen in Fig. 4.7 as overlapping circles.

The three approaches are often synergistic, each increasing the effectiveness of the others. For instance, consider the introduction of a programme aimed at reducing injury and death in road accidents through increased use of seat belts—an example of a prevention programme. This could be assisted by passing legislation to make seat belts compulsory (health protection) and by explaining the benefits of seat belt use to the public (health education).

Disease prevention is often described as comprising three levels of activity: primary, secondary, and tertiary prevention.

Primary, secondary, and tertiary prevention

Primary prevention

Primary prevention involves stopping a disease or condition from occurring in the first place. Examples in the field of child health include immunization, fluoridation of water to prevent dental decay, legislation aimed at preventing accidents (health protection), and the 'Back to Sleep' campaign to reduce cot death. Many health promotion interventions can also be seen as primary prevention measures, aiming to increase resistance to ill health and promote positive health—for example, healthy eating programmes which help prevent obesity and diabetes, or interventions to reduce the uptake of smoking among young people. Primary prevention is often aimed at a whole population, such as a community, school, or general practice caseload.

Secondary prevention

Secondary prevention refers to the early identification of disease or impairment, so that it can be reversed or its effects mitigated through treatment. Screening programmes are examples of secondary prevention, such as the neonatal blood spot ('Guthrie') test for congenital metabolic disorders including hypothyroidism (the impact of which can be all but eliminated by early intervention). Another example is interventions to prevent the recurrence of events or illnesses, including instituting child protection measures for abused children.

Tertiary prevention

Tertiary prevention involves slowing the progress and managing the consequences of established disease or disability, with the aim of alleviating its impact on the lives of the sufferer and his or her family. Examples include the use of inhalers to reduce the frequency and severity of a child's asthma attacks, supplying a wheelchair to a child with severe cerebral palsy to aid mobility, or teaching an adolescent with spina bifida self-catheterization to enable independent toileting.

Universal and targeted approaches

Whenever interventions are being considered, whether they are preventive or thera-peutic, some thought needs to be given to who should receive them. Some interven-tions, such as healthy eating advice, are appropriate for a whole population; others may apply only to some members—perhaps a particular age group (e.g. the child health immunization programme) or ethnic group (e.g. screening for thalassaemia or sickle cell disease). But we also need to consider the fact that interventions which could benefit everyone in the population to some extent may have greater advan-tages for some members than others: although increasing their levels of exercise would do everyone some good, for example, the health benefits are more marked for those who are sedentary than for those who already exercise regularly. Should we, then, be aiming interventions (and the limited resources available to support them) at those who have the greatest need, or who are at greatest risk? In some cases this approach is appropriate, but the argument is not as clear as one might first imagine.

In *The strategy of preventive medicine*, the late Geoffrey Rose argued that the population cannot be neatly divided into the sick and the healthy. For most diseases or health problems there is a continuum of severity rather than an absolute distinction between those with the disease and those without. The 'case definition' of a disease often involves a convenient, conventional, but more or less arbitrary cut off—of body mass index for obesity, blood glucose for diabetes mellitus, or peak flow for asthma, for example. This is even more pertinent when considering those at risk of disease. There is no clear dividing line between individuals 'at risk' and those 'not at risk' (see the detailed discussion of risk earlier in the chapter), even when we know that a particular indicator is an important risk factor. The risk of heart disease or stroke, for example, is not confined to those with the highest blood pressure; instead, there is a continuous distribution of risk throughout the entire population, with higher blood pressure tending to correlate to increasing risk, but some risk attached even to those with average or 'normal' blood pressure. In the maternal and child health setting, the same applies to defining those at risk of Down's syndrome, speech and language delay, emotional and behavioural problems, or child abuse.

There are good arguments both for universal approaches to health promotion and disease prevention, and approaches which target high risk groups. Much depends on the aim of the programme and the nature of the intervention.

In looking at the total 'burden' of a particular disease or condition within a population, it is important to consider the actual numbers of individuals at each level of risk. As Fig. 4.8 shows, for many risk factors there are usually relatively few individuals at the extreme end of the risk distribution, and increasing numbers as we move down through the spectrum.

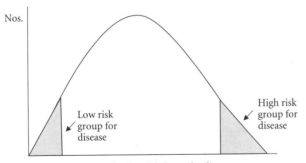

Fig. 4.8 Bell curve—low and high risk groups.

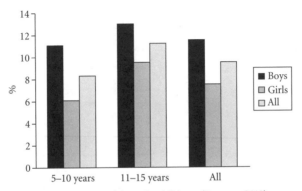

Fig. 4.9 Prevalence of behaviour problems in children. (Source: ONS)

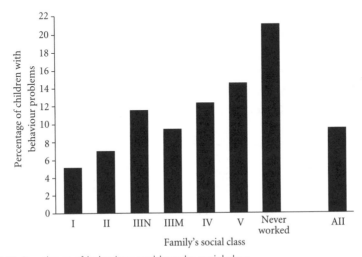

Fig. 4.10 Prevalence of behaviour problems by social class.

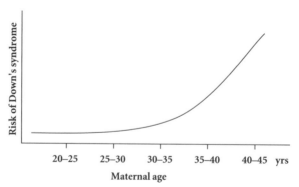

Fig. 4.11 Risk of Down's syndrome.

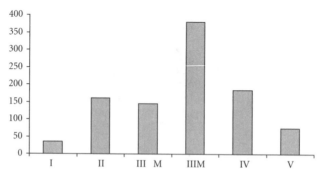

Fig. 4.12 No. of children (5–15 years) with behaviour problems in each social class in a population of 10,000. (Source: ONS)

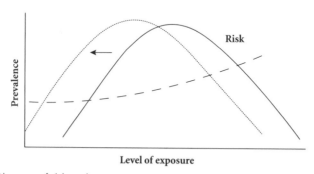

Fig. 4.13 Diagram of risk and exposure.

What implications does this have for disease prevention? Crucially, most cases of disease will occur among the many who are not at especially high risk, rather than among the few who are at very high risk. The majority of infants with Down's syndrome, for example, are born to mothers in younger age groups, although we know the individual risk is greater for the older mothers who make up a small proportion of the total pregnant population (Fig. 4.11).

Another example is illustrated in Fig. 4.9, 4.10 and 4.12. The prevalence of behaviour problems in 5–15 years-olds in the lowest social class is nearly three times that in the highest, but in any representative group of children the actual numbers affected are greatest in social class 3, which has a lower rate of problems but includes far more children. Interventions targeted at high risk groups (those from social class 5) are therefore bound to miss a high proportion of children with the problem.

Going back to the question posed earlier about whom interventions should be aimed at, it can be shown that in many situations a greater reduction in morbidity will be achieved by including the whole population and shifting the entire risk distribution downwards, rather than by attempting only to influence those at the upper end of the risk distribution. Examples might include child corporal punishment legislation in Scandinavia, which has substantially reduced exposure to physical violence across the entire child population, or school-based programmes to deliver free fruit to all children and thus increase average consumption of fruit and vegetables in the school-aged population. The impact of this kind of intervention is illustrated in Fig. 4.13: the broken curve shows the new lower distribution of exposure after a population-wide control measure which succeeds in shifting the entire risk distribution to the left. The total population risk (the area under the curve) is clearly much lower as a result—whereas merely eliminating the 'tail' at the top end of the risk distribution would have a much lesser impact.

It can be argued, therefore, that targeting interventions at those sections of the population with the highest risk, or the highest prevalence of problems, may not be the best way to reduce the burden of disease or problems in society as a whole. This is known as the **population paradox**. As Rose put it

> the visible tip of the iceberg of disease can be neither understood nor properly controlled if it is thought to constitute the entire problem.

This constitutes a strong argument, then, for universal interventions. The elimination of infectious diseases by the development of herd immunity is one good example of an effective population approach in which immunization of one group of people can protect others who cannot be immunized. Further arguments for the universal approach have been advanced by those interested in mental health promotion, since the mental health of the 'well' has an impact on the prevalence and severity of illness in the 'ill'. Racism, bullying, stigma, domestic violence, and child abuse are all important causes of mental health problems, but they are also indicators of less than optimal mental health among the perpetrators. Thus interventions to improve the mental health of the population as a whole arguably have an important role to play in reducing mental ill health amongst those most susceptible to it.

Reducing risk across a whole population can have a much greater impact than concentrating on high risk individuals. This is known as the population paradox.

On the other hand, the argument for a targeted strategy focussing on those at greater risk is that this approach is more efficient, yielding the most benefit given that resources are limited and may not stretch to cover a whole population. It is also the case that individuals who perceive themselves as being at lower risk are less likely to alter their behaviour and thus their risk profile, so that 'shifting the distribution downwards' may not be an easy outcome to achieve.

The efficiency argument in favour of targeted prevention has had a major impact on health visiting services, where caseloads are often 'profiled' according to various child and social risk factors, and divided into groups which receive different intensities of intervention according to their perceived level of need or risk. It is important here to point out the distinction between a *universal* and a *uniform* service. It is quite possible to provide universal coverage of a population in a preventive programme but to devote more time and resources to those in greatest need—and this is essentially what health visitors do in prioritizing their time.

It has been argued, moreover, that Rose's approach is not based on adequate scientific evidence. Also, risk can currently only be imprecisely defined according to broad bands or groups. Targeted interventions are clearly more appropriate, the argument goes, but we need a fuller understanding of the actual mechanisms of causation rather than descriptive statistical associations between risk and disease. If we could define individuals' risks of disease accurately, then interventions could be effectively and appropriately targeted. There is no doubt that many of the screening tools currently used for selecting the population to be 'targeted' (for example, assessment of mental health problems using the Edinburgh Postnatal Depression Scale) are imprecise, and may incorrectly classify individuals to receive—or not to receive—services.

There are persuasive arguments, then, in favour of both universal and targeted approaches to prevention. In practice, the choice of approach often reflects political or pragmatic considerations: the main aim of fluoridating water may be to reduce dental decay among disadvantaged children, but the most practical approach must be to treat the water supply for an entire area. Sometimes it is stigmatizing to select some individuals in a group to receive an intervention, and in order to improve uptake among those who most need it, it is better to offer a universal programme— health visiting services, as opposed to, e.g., social services involvement with a family. There is also an increasing recognition that the effectiveness of certain interventions is greatly increased by attempting to alter the behaviour or ethos of an entire group, via a 'settings' approach. This may involve promoting healthy schools, workplaces, even prisons or young offenders institutes: it brings us back to the earlier discussion about different levels for health promotion interventions, and the way in which they complement each other. It also reflects the fact that the social environment can be a powerful (positive or negative) influence on health, and that behaviour—especially among children and young people—is strongly influenced by the peer group.

Often, however, a combination of universal and targeted approaches is most appropriate. In seeking to reduce teenage pregnancy, we need to consider services for the whole teenage population (such as effective sex education programmes and easy availability of emergency contraception) and special interventions for those we know are at highest risk (including looked after children and those from disadvantaged backgrounds).

Finally, it is important to be clear about what a particular disease prevention programme hopes to achieve. One crucial distinction is between two different aims: a general decrease in morbidity across the whole population, or a reduction in health inequalities achieved by improving the health of the worst off and least healthy more than the better off and more healthy. It has become clear that general improvements in health often occur at the expense of widening gaps between the two extremes, and a targeted approach is often promoted as a way of reducing inequalities in health. The UK government has set a target for infant mortality which clearly sets the objective of reducing the difference between 'manual groups and the population as a whole'. Although many of the interventions and services which might contribute to this are universal (such as improvements in antenatal and neonatal care), others are aimed specifically at disadvantaged groups (such as 'Sure Start' schemes).

Screening

We have defined secondary prevention as the early identification of disease or impairment. There are two approaches to early diagnosis: one depends on prompt attention to the earliest symptoms of disease, the other to detection of latent or early disease in an apparently healthy, asymptomatic individual. The latter requires the administration of a *screening test*, usually as part of an organized screening programme, in order to identify individuals who:

- definitely have the disease or condition in question
- or, more commonly, have a result which indicates that they have a high chance of having the disease or condition

In the latter case, a second *diagnostic test* is required to confirm or refute the possible diagnosis. This might range from a relatively innocuous procedure, such as a more precise audiological test in the case of neonatal hearing screening, to an invasive procedure such as amniocentesis in the case of Down's syndrome screening.

> Screening tests and programmes aim to reduce risk—and thus prevent ill health—by detecting conditions at an early stage when interventions can be more effective.

In order for screening programmes to be appropriate and effective, certain conditions must be met. Wilson and Jungner first established a set of criteria against which proposed screening programmes could be assessed. A modified version of these is illustrated below, adapted by Hall and Michel specifically for neonatal screening programmes for liver disease and extra-hepatic biliary atresia, but equally applicable to other childhood screening programmes.

1. The condition should be an important public health problem as judged by the potential for heath gain achievable by early diagnosis.

2. There should be an accepted treatment or other beneficial intervention for patients with recognized or occult disease.

3. Facilities for diagnosis and treatment should be available and shown to be working effectively for classic cases of the condition in question.

4. There should be a latent or early symptomatic stage and the extent to which this can be recognized by parents and professionals should be known.

5. There should be a suitable test or examination. It should be simple, valid for the condition in question, reasonably priced, repeatable in different trials or circumstances, sensitive, specific. The test should be acceptable to the majority of the population.

6. The natural history of the condition and of conditions which may mimic it should be understood.

7. There should be an agreed definition of what is meant by a case of the target disorder; also an agreement as to (i) which other conditions are likely to be detected by the screening programme, (ii) whether their detection will be an advantage or a disadvantage.

8. Treatment at the early, latent, or presymptomatic phase should favourably influence prognosis, or improve outcome for the family as a whole.

9. The cost of screening should be economically balanced in relation to expenditure on the care and treatment of persons with the disorder and to medical care as a whole.

10. Case finding may need to be a continuous process and not a once and for all project, but there should be explicit justification for repeated screening procedures or stages.

More recently, the UK National Screening Committee has updated Wilson and Jungner's criteria to reflect a range of factors: recognition that screening is not infallible, that it can lead to harm as well as benefit (specifically in terms of its psychological impact, and in some cases the need for risky or invasive diagnostic procedures after a positive screening test), that it must be seen in the context of the entire range of service provision for the disease in question, and must be subject to strict quality controls to ensure it is effective. Their list of criteria is shown below.

UK National Screening Committee criteria

The condition

♦ The condition should be an important health problem.

♦ The epidemiology and natural history of the condition, including development from latent to declared disease, should be adequately understood and there should be a detectable risk factor, disease marker, latent period, or early symptomatic stage.

♦ All the cost effective primary prevention interventions should have been implemented as far as possible.

The test

◆ There should be a simple, safe, precise, and validated test.

◆ The distribution of the test values in the target population should be known and a suitable cut-off level defined.

◆ The test should be acceptable to the population.

◆ There should be an agreed policy on the further diagnostic investigation of individuals with a positive test result and on the choices available to those individuals.

The treatment

◆ There should be an effective treatment or intervention for patients identified through early detection, with evidence of early treatment leading to better outcomes than late treatment.

◆ There should be agreed evidence-based policies covering which individuals should be offered treatment and the appropriate treatment to be offered.

◆ Clinical management of the condition and patient outcomes should be optimized by all health care providers prior to participation in a screening programme.

The screening programme

◆ There should be evidence from high-quality randomized controlled trials that the screening programme is effective in reducing mortality or morbidity.

◆ There should be evidence that the complete screening programme (test, diagnostic procedures, treatment/intervention) is clinically, socially, and ethically acceptable to health professionals and the public.

◆ The benefit from the screening programme should outweigh the physical and psychological harm (caused by the test, diagnostic procedures, and treatment).

◆ The opportunity cost of the screening programme (including testing, diagnosis, and treatment) should be economically balanced in relation to expenditure on medical care as a whole.

◆ There should be a plan for managing and monitoring the screening programme and an agreed set of quality assurance standards.

◆ Adequate staffing and facilities for testing, diagnosis, treatment, and programme management should be available prior to the commencement of the screening programme.

◆ All other options for managing the condition should have been considered (e.g. improving treatment, providing other services).

Screening test properties

The ideal screening test has the ability to detect all those with the condition in question and exclude all those without it. This is rarely the case, and there are therefore almost invariably 'false positives' and 'false negatives' from the initial screening test—both of which have economic, psychological, and social costs attached. False positives (those with a positive screening test who turn out not to have the disease) are usually identified once the second diagnostic test has been applied, but false negatives (those with a negative result on the screening test, but who *do* have the disease) often do not emerge until later when the disease or condition reaches its overt stage. A useful framework for identifying false positives and negatives is given in the box below:

| | *Disease:* | |
Screening test:	Present	Absent
Positive	a	b
Negative	c	d

a True positive; *b* false positive; c false negative; *d* true negative

---

The performance of a screening test depends on the number of false positives and negatives it produces and is usually described in terms of its *sensitivity* and *specificity*—essentially, how good the test is at picking up cases and not picking up non-cases. Sensitivity refers to the proportion of cases of disease which are accurately detected by the test (and is lower if there are many false negatives); specificity refers to the proportion of those without the disease who are accurately detected by the test (and is lower if there are many false positives).

Another way of looking at a screening test's performance is to assess its *positive predictive value* and *negative predictive value*—or how useful a positive or negative test is in predicting the presence or absence of disease. Positive predictive value refers to the proportion of those testing positive who turn out to have the disease (lower if there are many false positives); negative predictive value refers to the proportion of those testing negative who turn out not to have the disease (lower if there are many false negatives). These concepts are defined mathematically in Table 4.7, using the letters from the box above.

The performance of a test is influenced not only by its own properties, but also by the prevalence of the condition in a particular population: although sensitivity and specificity depend only on the test, the positive and negative predictive values vary. Suppose the prevalence of Shergar's disease is 1% in a population of 100,000, and the sensitivity and specificity of the screening test designed to detect latent cases are both 90% (quite a reasonable assumption). There will be 1000 true cases, of which the test will detect 900; and there will be 99,000 healthy individuals of whom 9900 will also have positive results. Thus, out of a total of 10,800 positive results, only 900 will turn out to have Shergar's disease. The positive predictive value is therefore 900 ÷ 10,800 (a / a + b), which is 8.3%, and there will be 12 false positives for every true positive. If the prevalence is lower, say 0.1%, the positive predictive value will be 0.89%

Table 4.7 Mathematical definitions of sensitivity, specificity, positive and negative predictive values

Term	Definition	Formula
Sensitivity	The proportion of those with the condition *who test positive*	a / a + c
Specificity	Proportion without condition *who test negative*	d / b + d
Positive predictive value	Proportion with positive test *who have condition*	a / a + b
Negative predictive value	Proportion with negative test *who do not have condition*	d / c + d

and there will be 112 false positives picked up for every true positive. In addition, in either case 10% of those with Shergar's disease will be missed by the screening test and falsely reassured, although this will be a larger number when the prevalence is higher. The decision as to whether the cost in economic or social terms is acceptable is an important area for debate with the target population and their families or carers.

The performance of a screening test is influenced by its sensitivity and specificity, and also by the prevalence of the disease in the population.

It is clear that screening programmes are not infallible, and may in fact do more harm than good on balance if they are not carefully thought through. This is a concept which the general public finds hard to accept, especially when screening programmes are presented as beneficial services and there is a certain amount of pressure to accept testing. The National Screening Committee recognizes that screening programmes must be presented in a different way if they are to be acceptable and comprehensible to the population. Its second report stresses the importance of promoting individual choice about whether or not to undergo screening tests, and redefines screening as a risk reduction programme rather than as a reliable means of early diagnosis.

Advantages and disadvantages of screening programmes

A summary of the benefits and disadvantages of screening programmes is given in Table 4.8.

Table 4.8 Advantages and disadvantages of screening programmes

Benefits	Disadvantages
• Improved prognosis for some cases detected by screening	• Longer morbidity for cases whose prognosis is unaltered
• Less radical treatment which cures some early cases	• Possible overtreatment of questionable abnormalities
• Reassurance for those with true negative test results	• False reassurance for those with false negative results
• Lower resource costs for early treatment	• Anxiety and sometimes morbidity for those with false positive results
• May reduce overall incidence and prevalence of disease in population	• Hazard of screening test e.g. venepuncture, radiation
	• Resource costs: scarce resources diverted to screening programme
	• Unnecessary medical intervention for those with false positive results

Further reading

General texts

Blaxter, M. and Paterson, E. (1982). *Mothers and daughters: a three generational study of health attitutes and behaviour.* Heinemann, London.

Bradshaw, J. (1990). *Poverty and child health.* National Children's Bureau, London.

Detels, R., Holland, W., McKewan, J., and Omenn, G.S. (ed.) (1997). *Oxford textbook of public health.* Oxford University Press, Oxford.

Donaldson, L.J. and Donaldson, R.J. (2000). *Essential public health.* Petroc Press, Newbury.

Hill, A.B. (1965). The environment and disease: association or causation? *Proceedings of the Royal Society of Medicine* **58**: 295–300.

Last, J.M. (ed.) (1988). *A dictionary of epidemiology.* Oxford University Press, Oxford.

MacFarlane, A., Dunkley, R., and Wright, J. (1988). *Child public health training: a European perspective* (*see end of section for details). Public Health Resources Unit, Institute of Health Sciences, Oxford.

Mausner, J.S. and Kramer, S. (1985). *Epidemiology—an introductory text.* W.B. Saunders.

Rose, G. (1992). *The strategy of preventive medicine.* Oxford University Press, Oxford.

Rothman, K.J. (1986). *Modern epidemiology.* Little Brown, Boston.

Definitions of health

Pennington, J. (2002). Feeling happy and healthy, having fun and friends. Thesis submitted for degree of Doctor of Clinical Psychology. British Psychological Society.

Health promotion

Downie, R.S., Tannahill, C., and Tannahill, A. (1996). *Health promotion: models and values.* Oxford University Press, Oxford.

Earp, J.E. and Ennett, S.T. (1991). Conceptual models for health education research and practice. *Health Education Research*; 6:163–71.

Naidoo, J. and Wills, J. (1994). *Health promotion: disciplines and diversity.* Routledge, London.

Nutbeam, D. and Harris, E. (1999). *Theory in a nutshell: a guide to health promotion theory.* McGraw-Hill, Sydney.

Ottawa Charter for Health Promotion (1986). World Health Organisation, Geneva.

Prochaska, J.O., DiClemente, C.C., Velicer, W.F., and Rossi, J.S. (1993). Standardised, individualised, interactive and personalised self-help programs for smoking cessation. *Health Psychology*; 12:399–405.

Quah, S. (1985). The health belief model and preventive health behaviour in Singapore. *Social Science and Medicine*; 21:351–63.

Research Unit for Health and Behavioural Change (1989). *Changing the public health.* John Wiley, Chichester.

Advocacy

Hodgkin, R. (2000). *Advocating for children,* RCPCH London e-version on http://www.rcpch.ac.uk/publications.

Waterston, T. and Tonniges, T. (2001). Advocating for childrens health: a US and UK perspective. *Arch Dis Child*; 85:180–2.

Waterston, T. (2002). Advocacy for children. *Current Paediatrics*; 12:586–91.

Child health outcomes

Schmidt, L., Garrat, A., and Fitzpatrick, R. (2002). Child/parent assessed health outcome measures: a structured review. *Childcare health and development*; 28:237.

Social capital and inequalities

Coleman, J.S. (1990). *The foundations of social theory.* Harvard University Press, Cambridge MA.

Cooper, H., Arber, S., Fee, L., and Ginn, J. (1999). *The influence of social support and social capital on health. A review and analysis of British data.* Surrey Institute of Social Research. Health Education Authority, London.

Earls, F. and Carlson, M. (2001). The social ecology of child health and wellbeing. *Annual Review of Public Health*; 22:143–66.

Jarman, B. (1983). Identification of underprivileged areas. *BMJ*; 286:1705–9.

Kawachi, I. and Berman, L. (2000). Social cohesion, social capital and health. In *Social epidemiology* (ed. Berkman, L and Kawachi, I). Oxford University Press, Oxford.

Kawachi, I., Kennedy, B.P., Lochner, K., Prothrow–Stith, D. (1997). Social capital, income inequality and mortality. *American Journal of Public Health*; 879:1491–8.

Putnam, R. (2000). *Bowling alone.* Simon and Schuster, New York.

Putnam, R. (1993). *Making democracy work: civic traditions in modern Italy.* Princeton University Press, Princeton.

Rifkin, S. (1990). *Community participation in maternal and child health/family planning programmes.* World Health Organisation, Geneva.

Runyan, D.K., Hunter, W.M., and Amaya Jackson, L. (1998). Children who prosper in unfavorable environments: the relationship to social capital. *Pediatrics*; 101:12–18.

Sampson, R., Raudenbush, S., and Earls, F. (1997). Neighborhoods and violent crime: a multi-level study of collective efficacy. *Science*, 277:918–24.

Townsend, P., Philmore, P., and Beattie, A. (1998). *Health and deprivation: Inequality and the North*. Routledge, London.

Risk

Edwards, A.G.K. and Elwyn, G. (ed.) (2001). *Evidence based patient choice—inevitable or impossible?*, pp. 3–18. Oxford University Press, Oxford.

O'Connor, A., Fiset, V., Rosto, A. *et al.* (2002). *Decision aids for people facing health treatment or screening decisions. Cochrane Library Issue 1*. Update Software, Oxford.

Screening

First, second, and third reports of the National Screening Committee. Available at *www.nelh.org/screening*

Current UK health promotion programme – http://www.health-for-all-children.co.uk

Hall, D. and Elliman, D. (2003). *Health for all children* (4th edition). Oxford University Press, Oxford.

* **Results of a Delphi consultation in Europe on the subjects to be taught in child public health (APEE/ESSOP).**

Rank	Subjects to be taught at postgraduate level
1	Influences of social and environmental factors affecting peri-natal health
2	Evaluating effectiveness of screening and surveillance methods in childhood
3	Adolescent lifestyle issues
=4	Collaboration between services involved in child health
=4	Effective health promotion
6	Measurements of child health and quality of life
7	Appropriate services for disabled children other than medical ones
8	The consequences of childhood illness and disabilities within the child's social and financial context
9	Research methodologies relevant to children's health
10	Causes and prevention of mental illness
11	Educational influences on the health of children
12	Advocacy for child health issues
13	Quantitative and qualitative research methodologies as they relate to child health
14	Use of child health outcome indicators
15	Use of epidemiological studies to examine the aetiologies of childrens physical, mental, and emotional problems
=16	The settings of child health including schools, local communitites, cities
=16	Demographic trends in child health in Europe
18	How to put the UN convention into practice

19   UN convention as it applies to children with disability
20   Organizational model of primary, secondary, and tertiary care services, including effective management models
21   Adoption and fostering laws
22   Influences of television and media on child health and parenting
23   Communication systems within children's health services
24   Labour laws as they relate to children, including ethical issues concerning child rights and international differences

Chapter 5

Child health and adult health

History revisited

The belief that health in childhood is an important determinant of health in adulthood was widely held a century ago, and the particular vulnerability of infants and fetuses was well recognized. This belief contributed to the development of a number of the public health programmes described in Chapter 3 which aimed to enhance maternal, infant, and child health and welfare. The dramatic improvement in infant and child mortality rates that occurred during the last half of the nineteenth and first half of the twentieth century (see Chapter 3) fuelled the belief that child health was no longer a problem, and the focus of public health interest shifted to the newly emerging 'epidemics' of adult cardiovascular diseases and cancer. Recent developments in understanding the biology of mental and physical development, in the identification of childhood risk factors for adult disease, and in the importance of early care, are now rekindling the interest of policy makers in the health of children and allowing them to see that interventions to improve child health may be very important to the improvement of public health in general.

Different research paradigms

Our current understanding of the links between child and adult health is attributable to those in a range of academic disciplines who continued to research the childhood origins of adult disease during the period when most public health interest was focussed elsewhere. They include biologists and nutritionists interested in growth, development, and infectious diseases; social scientists and epidemiologists interested in the impact of social deprivation across generations; and child psychologists, psychiatrists, and psychotherapists interested in the impact of early care and relationships. Each of these groups has identified different factors in childhood that have an impact on health in adulthood, and each has favoured different explanations for the way in which the factors they identified impact on adult health.

Biological programming

The biologists have espoused the concept of biological programming. The belief that insults to health early in life can have an irreversible impact on health throughout life is well supported by observation, as is the idea that these insults may only matter during critical periods of human development. The impact of rubella infection on the fetus in the first trimester of pregnancy is a good example. This infection, which is relatively innocuous to human health at other times of life, can have a devastating and irreversible effect on the development of the cardiovascular and nervous systems of the fetus. Rubella immunization, first in teenage girls and now in one year olds in the combined MMR vaccine, is one of the many public health successes attributable to the biological sciences. It has led to the virtual elimination of disability caused by rubella infection. The studies of Nobel prize winners Hubert and Wiesel, demonstrating that the development of vision is dependent on the stimulus of light rays entering the eye during a critical period in the life of the kitten, is another good example, and one which has also had an important impact on clinical practice in child health.

> Biological programming—a biological stimulus (such as an infection or the lack of a key nutrient) at a critical period of development causes a lasting positive or negative effect on health.

Socio-economic circumstances

The social scientists and epidemiologists have focussed more on the explanatory paradigm of socio-economic circumstances, demonstrating that poverty and social deprivation in childhood have an impact on the risk of disease, not just in childhood, as we saw in Chapter 1, but throughout life. Those espousing this approach take a life course approach and suggest that exposures to inadequate socio-economic circumstances accumulate over time for three reasons. First, because one such experience predisposes the individual to experience another; second, because each experience has a damaging impact on the individual's resilience to other negative experiences; and third, because social resources and opportunities are constrained by various forms of social stratification and by social institutions (social patterning). These factors are said to prevent the development of 'health capital', which in turn leaves the individual vulnerable to a wide range of diseases throughout the course of their life.

Early care and nurture

Academics interested in the development of mental health and social well-being have shown that the quality of the relationship between babies and their carers has an important impact on the development of the capacity for emotional interaction with others and the capacity to manage or regulate emotions. These qualities are critical for the development of mental health in the positive sense and also affect the individual's capacity to form the sort of adult relationships which support health and well-being. These are described in Chapter 4, under the heading of 'social capital'.

Partly because such relationships protect against both mental and physical illness, and partly because continuing emotional distress has a detrimental impact on many biological systems, babies who are not cared for by nurturing adults are at increased risk of a wide range of adverse health outcomes in adulthood. Researchers working in this paradigm have shown that children are particularly vulnerable to lack of nurture in the first three years of life, but the effects of unhelpful parenting can be demonstrated in studies of children up to adolescence.

In the last ten years, this research has derived support from the observations of another group of biologists—developmental neuroscientists—who are now able to document the impact of nurture on brain growth and development in both animal and human studies.

Early care and nurture—the relationship between babies and their main carer (usually the mother) has a decisive and long-lasting impact on mental health, relationships, and the ability to learn. The 'prime time' for social and emotional development is in the first three years of life. Negative experiences or absence of appropriate stimulation at this time are more likely to have sustained and serious effects, but detrimental relationships later in childhood can also be damaging. Some of these effects can be reversed later in life.

Policy implications of the different paradigms

These three schools of thought suggest different public health approaches. Those who believe in programming would invest in nutritional and immunological support to mothers and children during pregnancy and infancy. Those who are concerned with the cumulative influences of social factors throughout life have the eradication of childhood poverty as their favoured intervention. Those who are concerned with the importance of nurture would put in place programmes for parents which enable them to care for their children in a more helpful way.

What emerges from an overview of the evidence presented by the three schools of thought, however, is that there is unlikely to be one single explanation for the impact of child health on adult health. The theories of these three groups are not mutually exclusive and it is likely that they all play a part. All three are also compatible with the belief that genetic susceptibility, which is not amenable to social, public health, or medical intervention, plays a part in causation. Each of the three paradigms is also compatible with the belief that threats to health in adulthood—such as violence, poverty, or everyday unhealthy lifestyles—have an impact on population health over and above that which has its origins in childhood.

The evidence base for biological programming
The Barker hypothesis

The concept of biological programming is currently being put forward as a mechanism to explain the strong and consistent relationship between birth weight and aspects of health in adult life. The most vociferous proponent of this school of thought is Barker, who hypothesizes that nutritional insults to the fetus during pregnancy determine vulnerability to cardiovascular disease in later life, and that these may be compounded by nutritional insults in the first year of life. His early studies were

Table 5.1 Death rates from coronary heart disease among 15,726 men and women according to birth weight

Birth weight in lbs (kg)	Standardized mortality ratio	Deaths (no.)
<5.5 (2.50)	100	57
Up to 6.5 (2.95)	81	137
Up to 7.5 (3.41)	80	298
Up to 8.5 (3.86)	74	289
Up to 9.5 (4.31)	55	103
>9.5 (4.31)	65	57
Total	74	941

(Source: Osmond, C., Barker, D.J.P., Winter, P.D. *et al*. *BMJ* (1993) **307**:1519–24, with permission from the BMJ Publishing Group.)

based on the archived records of health visitors in Hertfordshire and Sheffield in the early part of this century, and the linking of birth and early life records to death certificates. Many other studies in the UK, USA, Scandinavia, and developing countries have confirmed the association between birth weight and coronary heart disease mortality risk.

Together, these studies show a doubling of risk for babies weighing less than 5.5 lbs compared to those weighing 9.5 lbs, and a dose–response relationship. The hypothesis is supported by studies showing that the coronary heart disease risk factors, including hypertension, insulin resistance, and non-insulin dependent diabetes are also more common in those with low birth weight. The relationship between birth weight and blood pressure is held to be particularly strong. A body of evidence (not quite as strong as that for coronary heart disease) also links birth weight to stroke in later life. As stroke shares many risk factors with heart disease, this is not altogether surprising.

Barker's hypothesis that the mechanism is nutritional derives support from animal experiments. These show that under-nutrition *in utero* can lead to persisting changes in blood pressure, cholesterol metabolism, insulin response to glucose, and a range of other metabolic and immune processes known to be important in the development of cardiovascular disease in humans.

Criticisms of the Barker hypothesis

Growth in childhood, as opposed to growth *in utero* or in infancy, has also been shown to be strongly associated with coronary heart disease risk, suggesting that the impact is not confined to a critical period in pregnancy or the first year of life. However, a small number of studies have examined birth weight data, child height data, and final adult height data together, using regression analyses to adjust statistically for the potential confounding effects of adult health-related lifestyles and adult socio-economic status. These studies have shown that the birth weight/cardiovascular disease relationship remains significant, if attenuated, even when all these other factors have been taken into account, thus supporting Barker's belief in the importance of biological programming *in utero*.

Studies supporting the Barker hypothesis have been criticized on the grounds of publication bias—that is, that only studies in which a relationship has been found have been written up and submitted for publication. A recent meta-analysis carried out by Huxley of studies of the relationship between birth weight and blood pressure has demonstrated that the larger studies show smaller effects and that some very large studies from other research groups have not been able to corroborate Barker's findings.

While these studies have suggested that the impact of birth weight on cardiovascular disease risk may be smaller than previously supposed, it nonetheless seems likely that there is an epidemiological relationship between the two. The mechanisms involved in this relationship, however, are not well established. Studies set up by the Barker group to identify the specific nutritional deficiencies in pregnancy which might lead to low birth weight and cardiovascular disease risk in humans have failed to produce clear-cut findings.

Alternative, non-nutritional hypotheses to explain the relationship between birth weight and cardiovascular disease in adulthood suggest that birth weight is acting as a marker of socio-economic conditions, and that it is these, rather than the specific nutritional insults, which are responsible for adult disease risk. There is also a possibility that nurture plays an aetiological role in this process, through its capacity to prevent prolonged emotional distress. Studies (see, for example, Lou *et al.* 1994) have suggested that maternal stress in pregnancy is linked to low birth weight, and poverty and social deprivation are causes of maternal stress. The potential for emotional distress to inhibit growth later in childhood is recognized clinically in the phenomenon of psychosocial growth retardation.

Thus, both in pregnancy and in childhood, emotional distress appears to have the potential to interfere with growth. Through the mechanisms outlined later in this chapter, maternal distress (for example in the form of post-natal depression) creates distress in childhood, and distress in childhood persists into adulthood. Adult distress is a risk factor for cardiovascular disease. Emotional distress is therefore another potential confounding factor between poor socio-economic conditions, fetal and childhood growth, and adult cardiovascular disease. These different mechanisms are of course not mutually exclusive and all three may be acting together.

Respiratory disease

Respiratory diseases are caused by a complex interaction of infection, allergy, mucous secretion, and airways obstruction. Pollutants such as tobacco smoke also play an important role. Child health has been linked to adult respiratory health in a number of ways, and biological programming has been proposed as the mechanism for at least one of these relationships.

Historical cohort studies have provided evidence to link both infection and allergy development in childhood to respiratory health in adulthood. For example, there is growing, but incomplete, evidence that allergic sensitization (atopy), which is important in the development and prognosis of asthma, may be influenced by events during critical periods in infancy. This hypothesis centres on the belief that early exposure to infectious agents *protects* against the development of atopy. There may be a switching to alternative immunological pathways which is triggered by *non-exposure* to infectious agents.

The hypothesis is supported by the observation that children from large families and those from less affluent families are at reduced risk of developing atopic diseases such as hay fever and eczema. The evidence is less clear when it comes to determining the length and stage of the critical period if such a mechanism does exist.

Whilst exposure to infectious agents in general early in childhood has been proposed as protective against some chest disease, chest infections in childhood have been shown to increase the risk of productive cough, wheeze, and impaired ventilatory function in adulthood. This relationship does not seem to be confined, as was first suggested, to a particular period of childhood in the way that would be expected if biological programming was operating.

The detrimental impact on the respiratory system of exposure to tobacco smoke does not show a critical period effect, operating instead throughout childhood, starting with the impact of exposure to 'passive smoke' *in utero*. As well as its influence on birth weight, this increases the risk of chest infection in childhood. Passive smoking in childhood also increases the risk of chest infections and plays a role in the aetiology of childhood asthma. Through the link between childhood chest infection and adult respiratory disease, this exposure has an influence on health in adulthood. As yet, the evidence suggesting that respiratory health in adulthood may be programmed by infections or other exposure in infancy is circumstantial and does not propose any obvious interventions. In contrast, the evidence suggesting that the inhalation of tobacco smoke at any time in pregnancy and childhood leads to respiratory problems in both childhood and adulthood is strong, and has much clearer implications for intervention.

Cognitive development

A nutritional programming hypothesis has also been put forward to explain the observation that preterm delivery appears to have an impact on cognitive development. Early nutritional intervention in preterm babies, using breast milk as opposed to artificial alternatives, results in significant improvements in the cognitive development of children at eight years. The fact that the relationship between preterm delivery and cognitive development can be reversed by breast milk in very early life provides evidence that nutritional inadequacy very early in life can influence mental performance in later years. Longer term follow-up studies will be needed to demonstrate that this effect is carried through to adulthood, but there are many studies showing that educational performance at eight years predicts educational achievement in late adolescence and that this in turn predicts employment prospects in adulthood. These studies do not of themselves demonstrate a critical period because they do not rule out the potential impact of nutrition on cognitive development late in childhood.

Summary: biological programming

♦ Biological programming has been proposed as a factor contributing to the aetiology of cardiovascular disease, respiratory disease, and cognitive development.

♦ Early interventions, for example to improve the diet of pregnant women and babies, might alter the course of development and improve the health of the growing child and adult.

♦ The specific nutritional factors which might explain these relationships have yet to be identified. There are no intervention studies to support the belief that dietary changes in pregnancy or infancy could affect cardiovascular disease risk in adulthood. Nor have studies on programming in respiratory disease yet provided potential interventions for testing.

The evidence base for the impact of socio-economic circumstances

Social scientists and epidemiologists have demonstrated, in numerous studies dating back over many years, that socio-economic conditions in childhood have an influence on health in adult life. Fig. 5.1 illustrates how survival in successive generations has improved over the last 150 years as socio-economic circumstances have improved. These are logarithmic plots showing the change in survival of successive cohorts whose year of birth is on the horizontal axis. They show very clearly the dramatic impact of improving socioeconomic circumstances on child health (illustrated by the steep decline in mortality in the 10–14 year age group). The impact on mortality in older age groups is much smaller. (see also Fig. 3.5, p. 95)

Two main mechanisms have been postulated to account for the observed link between socio-economic conditions in childhood and health in adulthood:

♦ socio-economic factors impact on health in childhood, and children with poor health grow up to be adults with poor health

♦ social inequality persists over the life course and it is poverty in adulthood that has a deleterious impact on health

These two mechanisms are explored further below.

The impact of social inequality on health in childhood

The numerous ways in which poverty affects health in childhood have been reviewed in Chapter 1 and these have an impact on both health and social position in adulthood. For example, disability (congenital and acquired) and infectious diseases are more common in lower socio-economic groups, and both, possibly through their impact on schooling, increase the chance of adult unemployment, which is in turn associated with ill health. The risk of injury is greatly increased for children living in deprived circumstances and injury is an important cause of disability in young

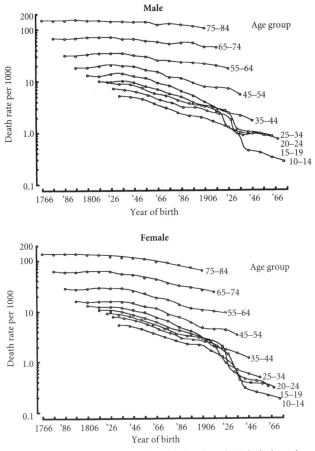

Fig. 5.1 Changes in generation mortality (England and Wales), based on age-specific death rates 1841–1990. (Source: Kuh, D., Power, C., Blane, D., and Hartley, M. (1997). *A life course approach to chronic disease epidemiology*. Oxford University Press, Oxford.)

adults. The diets of children living in poverty are less nutritious than those of children from other social groups.

Growth at all stages of childhood is influenced by socio-economic position, with children from more affluent backgrounds being taller. Childhood height predicts adult height, and adult height is an important predictor both of disease and of social position. Men who are tall have a greater chance of upward social mobility. For women, it is the influence of low socio-economic status on obesity that has a greater influence. Obese women have a reduced chance of marrying up the social scale and thus increasing their life chances, and obesity itself is an important risk factor for disease.

Girls who were born poor have an increased risk of teenage pregnancy, and this is strongly associated with childhood poverty. They are also at greater risk of poor reproductive experience. The chances of a teenager starting to smoke are influenced by whether their parents smoke, and smoking is much more common in lower social groups. Low socio-economic status increases the risk of poor family functioning, parental conflict, and adverse parenting styles, which reduce the chances of a child developing good social skills and increase the risk of anti-social behaviour and school drop-out. These all increase the likelihood of the adoption of unhealthy lifestyles and substance misuse in adolescence, reduce the chance of forming supportive interpersonal relationships and gaining secure employment in adulthood, and increase the chance of delinquency and crime.

Thus a range of social and environmental factors can impact on different aspects of children's health and many of these health problems have implications for adult health. Figure 5.2 illustrates the effects of socio-economic and demographic influences in childhood on later adult health morbidity. It shows that three important childhood socio-economic factors—poverty, large family size, and family breakdown—all independently increase the odds of mental and physical health problems in adulthood, after taking age, sex, and adult social class into account. Interestingly, this study also suggests that family conflict (see Chapter 1) is a more important predictor than any of these three socio-economic indicators.

Persistence of social inequality

An adverse social environment in childhood predisposes to an adverse social environment in adulthood, and there are a very large number of studies showing that such circumstances in adulthood—poverty, unemployment, and poor work environment in particular—increase the risk of ill health. The 1946 and 1958 birth cohort studies both demonstrate that those born into poor social backgrounds were more likely to be poor themselves in adulthood.

Having an unemployed father at the age of 16 doubles the risk of a man experiencing unemployment in adulthood, and long-term unemployment of the father at age 16 increases the risk five-fold. In this way cycles of social disadvantage are created, with each generation at increased risk of being exposed to the same detrimental social circumstances as the previous generation. One of the intervening factors accounting

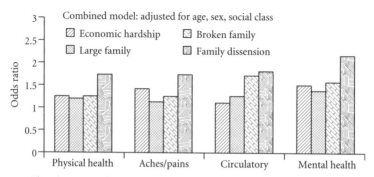

Fig. 5.2 The impact of childhood living conditions on health in adulthood. (Source: Lundberg (1993). *Soc Sci Med*; **36**:1047–52, permission sought.)

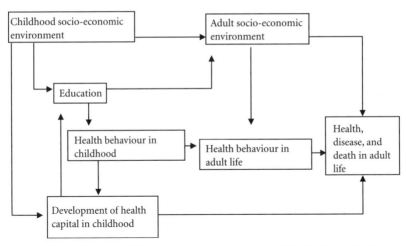

Fig. 5.3 Pathways between childhood and adult health. (From Kuh, D., Power, C., Blane, D., and Hartley M. (1997). Social pathways between childhood and adult health. In *A life course approach to chronic disease epidemiology* (ed. Kuh, D. and Ben-Shlomo, Y.). Oxford University Press, Oxford.)

for this social continuity may be educational achievement. Family background has an influence on educational attainment, with low socio-economic status predicting educational failure. Educational attainment has an influence on adult income and occupation. Qualifications on leaving school can be shown to predict adult mortality, blood pressure, and self-rated health, and poor educational attainment earlier in school life predicts the adoption of unhealthy lifestyles.

Studies which have tried to unravel the separate effects of education and other aspects of social deprivation in childhood, on health in adulthood have, however, failed to show that educational under-achievement can account for the full effect of childhood social deprivation on adult health.

Strategies for prevention

These two groups of studies together provide unequivocal evidence that socio-economic factors operating in childhood have an influence on health in adulthood. However, they also give rise to questions, important in determining strategies for prevention, as to whether it is the experience of adverse social circumstances in adulthood or childhood that matter most. Studies which have tried to tease this out have demonstrated an independent impact of both, suggesting an ongoing vulnerability attributable to poor social circumstances in childhood coupled with increased risks attributable to exposure in adulthood. Those living in poor socio-economic circumstances throughout life have the poorest health, at least as measured by coronary heart disease risk.

Whilst there have been no controlled studies of income redistribution, observation of the impact of changing patterns of childhood poverty on infant and childhood mortality support the proposal that reduction in childhood poverty would have an important impact on child and adult health. A number of studies have examined strategies for preventing the health consequences of childhood social deprivation and there is evidence that these can be effective. Early education interventions such as 'Head Start' in the USA, which support the cognitive and social development of children through well-resourced day care, are highly cost-effective in mitigating the effects of social disadvantage. Infant mental health interventions (see Chapter 7) can enhance resilience to the damaging effects of poverty and deprivation. These may increase parents' capacity to nurture their babies, increase their confidence as parents, and encourage personal development, leading to greater employment opportunities. All these approaches may be combined in a single programme with the potential for synergistic effects. A range of studies indicate that it is possible to have a positive impact on injury risk in deprived communities.

Summary: socio-economic circumstances

+ There is robust evidence to show that socio-economic circumstances in childhood have an effect on health in adulthood.

+ Two different mechanisms have been explored. The first shows that socio-economic circumstances impact on child health directly and that these effects track through into adulthood; the second, that socio-economic circumstances in childhood are predictive of socio-economic circumstances in adulthood and that these have an impact on adult health.

+ There is evidence that both mechanisms operate. Those living in poor socio-economic circumstances throughout life have the poorest health through a cumulative effect on health risk. The findings are more in keeping with a life course effect than with programming.

+ Observation of trends in poverty and childhood mortality suggests that income redistribution programmes would improve both child and adult health.

The evidence base for early care and nurture

Contributions to the literature showing that early care and nurture has an impact on health in adulthood have been made from several different academic groups. One group has a psychotherapeutic orientation and takes its lead from John Bowlby. He studied children in care, documenting the progression to profoundly disturbed mental health and interpersonal relationships in adulthood of those who were deprived of a caring relationship with an adult during the early period of their lives. Bowlby's research was seized on in the post-war period by policy makers concerned about unemployment amongst men being decommissioned from the armed forces. They used his findings to make the case that mothers should stay at home to care for their children rather than participating in the labour force, thus freeing up jobs for ex-soldiers.

This distortion of Bowlby's recommendations brought his theories into disrepute. In spite of this, his writings have had an enduring impact on paediatric practice, leading to changes in hospital policies which formerly separated children from their parents. They have also influenced child psychiatrists, who have continued to research the importance for mental health and relationships of the parent–child relationship, and the phenomenon of attachment or bonding of mother and baby, during the last fifty years. Donald Winnicott, in particular, built on and developed Bowlby's work, making careful observations of mother–infant relationships.

Attachment, conflict, abuse, and discipline

The impact of early relationships on children's emotional and social development was outlined in Chapter 1. Children who develop mental health problems and difficulties with peer relationships as a consequence of not experiencing attuned, sensitive parenting are at high risk of growing up to be adults with mental illness, personality disorder, drug and alcohol misuse, and problems with relationships. Up to half of all babies can be shown in some studies to have less than optimal attachment patterns.

Chapter 1 also outlined the importance of appropriate parenting in later childhood (including warmth, supervision, and positive discipline) for child development. It described the detrimental effects of family conflict, domestic violence, and child abuse on emotional and social development, particularly conduct disorder and antisocial behaviour. A large number of studies carried out over a long period of time attest to the fact that children with such mental health problems grow up to be adults with antisocial behaviour. These children are at high risk, as adults, of:

- criminality and imprisonment
- delinquency, violence, and antisocial behaviour
- depression and anxiety
- drug and alcohol misuse
- forming destructive relationships and experiencing marital breakdown.

The long-term impact of abuse, particularly sexual abuse, on mental health has been most studied in women, where it has been shown to be an important risk factor for depression and drug misuse in adulthood. The development of post-traumatic stress disorder in childhood as a consequence of abuse represents one possible biological mechanism.

Adults with antisocial behaviour are more likely to be convicted of both violent and non-violent crimes, and they are less likely to be able to hold down a job. They are more likely to be violent towards their spouses and children, and to have a detrimental effect on the 'social capital' of communities in which they end up living. One of the features of communities with high social capital is that they show norms of social trust, a commodity that is scarce in places with high crime rates. As we have seen in Chapter 4, social capital is an important determinant of adult health. People living in communities with high social capital live longer than those in communities where there is little. Through this link, therefore, poor parenting experienced by some children can have important detrimental effects, when both reach adulthood, on the health of other children.

The development of the emotional brain and neurohumoral mechanisms

Recent developments in brain imaging—functional magnetic resonance imaging (MRI), positron emission topography, and non-invasive electro-encephalographic (EEG) recording—have enabled neuroscientists to study brain development in the human infant. These techniques, together with animal studies, have revolutionionized our understanding of brain development. Brain growth is at is its peak in the first three years of life, but is dependent on optimum environmental conditions. At three years of age, the infant brain has twice the number of synapses of the adult brain. Subsequent brain development is use-dependent. Pathways that are well used become protected, whereas those that are not used are pruned. Rats raised in enriched environments have 25% more synaptic connections as adults than those raised in sparse environments.

A number of studies, some in animals and some in humans, have shown that the development of the emotional brain is critically dependent on nurturing care in the very early years. The prefrontal cortex, hippocampus and amygdala are poorly developed in babies who have not received such care. Observation of the behaviour of animals who have been deprived of sensitive nurturing care in early life and of infants who have lived in fear of abandonment, humiliation or physical attack suggest that they are 'hard wired' in later life to anticipate threatening relationships with others. The dominance of such pathways puts people at risk of mental illness, makes learning difficult and creates the expectation that relationships with others will be harmful. In contrast, infants who have received nurturing care are more likely to anticipate supportive, encouraging relationships and to behave accordingly.

Studies on different aspects of brain development—cognitive, sensory, and emotional—suggest that whilst there are no critical periods there are 'prime times' for optimal development. Thus the optimal time for language development is in the preschool period. They also suggest that brain development is remarkably plastic and that it is possible for functions which have not developed at the prime time to develop later. It is however more difficult for them to do so, and optimum conditions are required. The prime time for the development of the parts of the brain involved in emotion appears to be the first three years of life. The potential for neural development or learning to continue throughout life, and the ability of one part of the brain to support deficient functioning in another (neural plasticity) means that some damaging neural pathways developed during childhood can be reversed later in life. Long-term follow-up studies of damaged children suggest, however, that in the absence of intervention this does not normally happen, and that children who grow up with parents who cannot provide supportive care are at increased risk in adulthood of a wide range of mental and physical health problems.

Recent developments in neuroscience have revolutionized our understanding of the development of the brain and shown the vital role that early nurture and care play in this process.

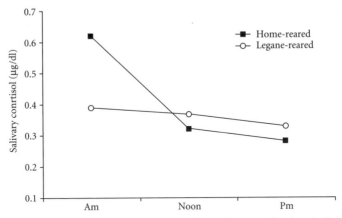

Fig. 5.4 Loss of normal circadian salivary cortisol measurements in chronically stressed children in Romanian orphanages (Leganes). (Source: Carlson, M. and Earls, F. (1997). Psychological and neuroendocrinological sequelae of early social deprivation in institutionalised children in Romania. *Annals of New York Academy of Sciences*; **807**:419–28, permission sought.)

Secure attachment is therefore necessary for the normal development of the emotional brain, and it also appears to be necessary for the development of a normal hypothalamic–pituitary response to stress. Babies receiving warm nurturing care are less inclined to respond to stress by producing cortisol and they can more rapidly and efficiently turn off this response. High corticotrophin releasing hormone (CRH) levels are associated with increased neuronal cell death, and this may be of particular significance in the young and rapidly developing infant brain. Children with chronically high levels of cortisol are more likely to show developmental delay. Studies of children in Romanian orphanages and others who have been subjected to chronic stress and maltreatment have shown blunting of the normal cortisol biorhythm. This early 'resetting' of the hypothalamic–pituitary–adrenal system represents a possible mechanism through which chronic hypocortisolism of adult-hood develops. The latter has been linked to increased risk of psychological and physical morbidity.

Links to physical health in adulthood

Literature is now emerging to show that aspects of the parent–child relationship predict physical health in adulthood. Students at Harvard University in the USA who did not feel close to and respect their parents have been shown to be at increased risk of a range of common diseases in adulthood, including heart disease and musculoskeletal disease. Swedish adults who reported experiencing family conflict

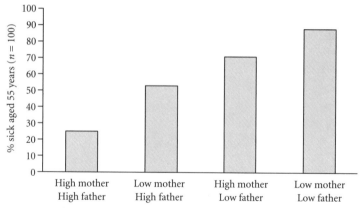

Fig. 5.5 Parental caring and health status in midlife. (Drawn from data presented in Russek and Schwartz (1997). *Psychosomatic Medicine*; **59**:144–9, permission sought.)

in childhood have also been shown to be at increased risk of these common adult health problems (see Fig. 5.2, p. 162).

Such long-term follow-up studies are very rare, but they confirm the possibility that the various neurobiological mechanisms demonstrable in early life could be taking their toll on long-term health. They are also important because they demonstrate the impact of parenting in families who are not suffering from deprivation. There is no doubt that poor social circumstances make supportive and enabling parenting less easy, and there is also no doubt that parenting which is unhelpful to social and emotional development is more common in families living in deprived social circumstances. Studies such as those carried out on the Harvard students, however, suggest that socio-economic factors are not the *cause* of parenting which is damaging to health and development.

Intervention studies

A range of interventions have been developed to promote maternal sensitivity and attunement, and to increase parents' confidence and parenting skills. These are described in more detail in Chapter 7. Many of these interventions are effective in improving emotional and social development and peer interaction, and in reducing delinquency and violence in later life. It is also possible to work with children in day care and nurseries and compensate for unhelpful parenting. Studies suggest that such programmes can deliver improvement in the health of parents as well as that of their children. They appear to mitigate the deleterious effects of social disadvantage and have the potential to protect against susceptibility to a wide range of diseases in adulthood. Such studies have also shown that it is possible to improve the attitudes and beliefs which predict abuse, and to improve a range of child health outcomes including injury. However, they have yet to demonstrate a reduction in prosecuted cases of abuse, probably because of the difficulty of measuring abuse and bias in ascertainment of cases.

Summary: early care and nurture

- When infants and children are cared for by adults who support them when they feel threatened, encourage the development of their autonomy, and who do not themselves present a threat, they seem to develop neural pathways which anticipate such positive relationships with others and which allow opportunity for creativity and learning.

- Infants and children who live in fear of abandonment, humiliation, or physical attack seem to develop very different pathways—ones that are geared to dealing with threat.

- The dominance of such pathways makes learning difficult and creates the expectation that relationships with others will be harmful. Children such as these are at high risk of adult criminality and violence, depression, anxiety, drug and alcohol misuse, and personality disorder. They tend to form destructive interpersonal relationships.

- Because of the effect they have on social capital, such individuals can have an negative impact on the health of other members of communities.

- Nurturing care appears necessary for a normal hypothalamic–pituitary response to stress. The resetting of this response in children who live with chronic stress represents a possible mechanism for deleterious effects on physical and mental health.

- Longitudinal studies confirm lack of nurturing care in childhood to be predictive of both poor mental and physical health in adulthood. Intervention can be successful in enabling parents to change the way they parent.

Bringing it all together

The evidence base in support of the early care and nurture school of thought is strong and diverse, including both epidemiological and intervention studies published over a long time span. It is interesting, therefore, to consider why this school has, until recently, had such a minor influence on clinical, public health, academic, and political thinking. One of the problems may be that understanding of the mechanisms which underpin this theory has, until recently, depended on a knowledge of the psychology and psychotherapy literature with which few clinicians, public health practitioners, epidemiologists, and policy makers are familiar. The studies of the psychoneuroimmunologists and developmental neuroscientists are important in this respect, demonstrating the biological mechanisms that underpin the conclusions psychologists and psychotherapists have drawn from their observational studies.

Combining the knowledge bases of all three schools of thought and developing social policy which takes account of all three could have an important effect on public health. The impact that such policies could have on health in both adulthood and childhood could be as great as that delivered by the public health reforms of the last century. Although it is not yet clear which aspects of nutrition are especially important, good nutrition for pregnant women, infants, and children is very likely to have a beneficial impact on children's development. The development of social policy which makes the job of parenting easier and abolishes the stresses created by parenting in poverty would have an important effect on child and adult health. And finally, provision of programmes for parents which enable them to develop sensitivity towards their babies, to increase their respect for their children's autonomy, and to master the skills of positive discipline would gradually have an independent impact on very many aspects of child and adult health.

Further reading

(See also Chapters 1 and 7 for further reading on issues mentioned here but covered in more detail in these chapters.)

Anisman, H., Zaharia, M.D., Meaney, M.J., and Merali, Z. (1998). Do early-life events permanently alter behavioral and hormonal responses to stressors? *International Journal of Developmental Neuroscience;* 16(3/4):149–64.

Barker, D.J.P. (1998). *Mothers, babies and health in later life.* Churchill Livingstone, Edinburgh.

Bowlby, J. (1957). *Childcare and the growth of love.* Pelican Books, Middlesex. (Also Penguin, 1980).

British Medical Association (1999). (1) Emotional and behavioural problems. (2) Fetal origins of adult diseases. (3) Inequalities in child health. In *Growing up in Britain: ensuring a healthy future for our children. A study of 0–5 year olds.* British Medical Association, London.

Committee on Integrating the Science of Early Childhood Development (2000). (1) Nurturing Relationships. (2) Inequalities in child health. In *From neurons to neighborhoods: the science of early childhood development.* National Academy Press, Washington DC.

Davey Smith, G. (1997). Socio-economic differentials. In *A life course approach to chronic disease epidemiology* (ed. Kuh, D. and Ben–Shlomo, Y.). Oxford University Press, Oxford.

Gunnar, M.R. (1996). *Quality of care and buffering of stress physiology. Its potential in protecting the developing human brain.* University of Minnesota Institute of Child Development.

Heim, C., Ehlert, U., and Hellhammer, D.H. (2000). The potential role of hypocortisolism in the pathophysiology of stress-related bodily disorders. *Psychoneuro-endocrinology.* 25:1–35.

Huxley, R., Neil, A., and Collins, R. (2002). Unravelling the 'fetal origins' hypothesis: is there really an inverse association between birth weight and blood pressure? *Lancet.* 360:659–65.

Kuh, D., Power, C., Blane, D., and Bartley, M. (1997). Social pathways between childhood and adult health. In *A life course approach to chronic disease epidemiology* (ed. Kuh, D. and Ben–Shlomo, Y.) Oxford University Press, Oxford.

Ladd, C.O., Owens, M.J., and Nemeroff, C.B. (1996). Persistent changes in corticotropin-releasing factor neuronal systems induced by maternal deprivation. *Endocrinology.;* 137:1212–18.

Lou, H.C., Hansen, D., Nordentoft, M. *et al.* (1994). Prenatal stressors of human life affect fetal brain development. *Developmental Medicine and Child Neurology.* 6:826–32.

Lucas, A., Morley, R., Cole, T.J., Lister, G., and Leeson–Payne, C. (1992). Breast milk and subsequent intelligence quotient in children born preterm. *Lancet;* 339:261–4.

Patterson, G.R. (1989). A developmental perspective on antisocial behaviour. *American Psychologist;* 44:329–35.

Perry, B.D. (1994). Neurobiological sequelae of childhood trauma: PTSD in children. In *Catecholamine function in PTSD* (ed. Murberg, M.). American Psychiatric Press, Washington DC.

Perry, I.J. (1997). Fetal growth and development: the role of nutrition and other factors. In *A life course approach to chronic disease epidemiology* (ed. Kuh, D. and Ben–Shlomo, Y.) Oxford University Press, Oxford.

Plotsky, P.M. and Meaney, M.J. (1993). Early postnatal experience alters hypothalamic corticotropin-releasing factor (CRF) mRNA, median eminence CRF content and stress-induced release in adult rats. *Molecular Brain Research;* 18:195–200.

Robins, L.S. and Price, R.K. (1991). Adult disorders predicted by childhood conduct problems: results from NIMH epidemiologic catchment population. *Psychiatry.* 54:116–32.

Shore, R. (1997). *Rethinking the brain. New insights into early development.* Families and Work Institute, New York.

Stewart–Brown, S. (2000). Parenting, well-being, health and disease. In *Developing children's emotional well-being* (ed. Buchanan, A. and Hudson, B.) Oxford University Press, Oxford.

Strachan, D.P. (1997). Respiratory and allergic disease. In *A life course approach to chronic disease epidemiology* (ed. Kuh, D. and Ben–Shlomo, Y.) Oxford University Press, Oxford.

Suomi, S.J. (1997). Early determinants of behaviour: evidence from primate studies. *British Medical Bulletin;* 53:170–84.

Chapter 6

Techniques and resources for child public health practice

Community diagnosis

The practice of public health involves a focus on populations rather than individuals. The size and type of population can vary enormously: public health professionals can and do operate at international, national, regional, district, and local community level, with homogeneous and heterogeneous populations whose health, lives, and socio-economic circumstances span a wide range. There are clearly practical differences between projects focussed at national and local level, and between work in countries with very different infrastructure and health problems, but the principles of public health practice are similar whatever the size and nature of the population, and certain tools and techniques are fundamental to everyone working in the field. Although much of this book assumes a focus at the level of a primary care organization in a developed country such as the UK, the approaches described can be generalized to any setting.

> Public health involves a focus on populations rather than individuals, but—just as in clinical practice—the first step is to identify the problems to be addressed by defining and assessing health needs.

For any public health project or programme, the first step is to identify the problems to be addressed by defining and assessing the health needs of a population. In the UK, Health Improvement and Modernization Programmes (HIMPs) drawn up by health care providers and commissioners in partnership with other key players such as local government have been used to formulate local health policy. One of the main prerequisites for the development of a HIMP is the comprehensive assessment of the health and social needs of the local population—essentially, making a community diagnosis. This chapter describes some of the tools used in child public health practice which enable a community diagnosis (also known as a health needs assessment) to be formulated.

The diagnostic process has many parallels in clinical and public health practice. The triad of history taking, physical examination, and investigations make up the cornerstone of clinical activity in response to a patient presenting with a 'problem'. In making a 'community diagnosis', we are applying similar processes of listening to the population, observing the population, and carrying out special investigations with a view to better understanding of the issues or problems presented (see Table 6.1).

Table 6.1 Clinical and community diagnosis

	Clinical diagnosis	**Community diagnosis**
History	Symptoms, concerns, systems review, family and social, medications, allergy, etc	Concerns of local people and professionals Press reports of health issues Rapid appraisal needs assessment
Examination	Looking, feeling, listening	Examination of local and national statistics, local government reports, annual report of the director of public health, condition-based registers
Investigation	X-rays, blood tests, case conference	Surveys, case control or cross-sectional studies, geographical mapping

The analogy can be taken further. At both the individual and the population level, there are frequently multiple, often inter-related problems to be found rather than a single diagnosis, and the clinician or public health professional may need to prioritize in deciding which are important, and which to tackle first. The views of the patient/population are vital in reaching such a decision, and imposing the paternalistic judgement of a professional about 'what needs treating' may be inappropriate in both cases. Perhaps most importantly, the purpose of making a diagnosis in either situation is to move on to action, with a view to resolving or alleviating the problem which has been presented, and the patient population should wherever possible be an equal partner in that process.

> In public health practice, as in clinical practice, there are often several problems rather than a single diagnosis. Public health professionals, in conjunction with other professionals and local communities, need to decide which are priorities for action.

Some types of 'therapeutic activity' which are undertaken by a public health practitioner have already been touched on in earlier chapters (for example, health promotion and disease prevention, community development work, advocacy, and screening), and others (such as the development and implementation of health policy and strategies) will be explored in the final chapter. These are often less clear-cut than the clinical equivalents of treatment by medication, surgical intervention, or reassurance, and they invariably involve more players even than the modern multidisciplinary clinical team. However, there are still many similarities. At both the individual patient and community level trust, mutual respect, and fairness are crucial, together with a focus on producing a solution to the presenting 'problem'.

Finally, just as a good clinician will follow up his or her patient to assess the outcome of their treatment and the success of the therapeutic encounter as a whole—and to identify early the development of further complications or new problems—so the public health practitioner should always evaluate the outcome of any public health intervention or programme, and continue to reassess the situation to ensure that improvements have been maintained and any input continues to be appropriate and useful. The audit cycle is relevant to both situations, as are the principles of clinical governance and responsibility for the quality of the service provided.

One of the public health 'interventions' which may follow health needs assessment is the development or reconfiguration of local health (or social care) services to ensure that service provision reflects local need as far as possible. As in clinical practice, deciding what to do with the 'diagnosis' is often not a straightforward matter. It usually involves a stage of reflection and prioritization, balancing the relative significance of different problems—and different perspectives.

Consider, for example, the kind of problem lists which may emerge from the diagnostic process for a child with multiple disabilities on the one hand and a primary care organization's assessment of children's needs in its patch on the other. For the individual child, the list might include the improvement of mobility, the management of feeding, deteriorating control of epileptic fits, the development of contractures, and the fact that his parents are having increasing difficulty in coping physically as he grows. The child's dearest wish might be for a better wheelchair which would allow him to move around the school playground more easily and therefore integrate better with his peers. For the parents, overnight respite care a couple of nights a week might be the top priority. From the perspective of the medical team, referral to a surgeon for assessment of his contractures might be on the action list. His teachers might be pressing for adjustment of his anti-epileptic medication because they are having difficulty coping with fits in school. The social worker might be most concerned about behaviour problems in a younger sibling who has been receiving less attention lately and tensions in the parents' marriage, and might feel referral to a family centre is the most urgent need.

For the primary care organization, the problem list may include a shortage of nursing staff on the acute wards which means beds are currently closed, an increasing number of children with complex needs being placed (expensively) out of the area because of difficulty arranging appropriate educational provision for them locally, long waiting lists for child psychiatric assessment, a rising tide of substance misuse in local schools, the lack of community speech and language therapists, and a crisis of morale among health visitors due to reorganization of the service and conflicting priorities for their limited time. National targets, pressure points in services, and changes in demography and morbidity will all have to be taken into account. Again, different individuals and organizations may have a very different view of what matters most. It is clear that acute and community staff, parents and young people, teachers, social workers, community nurses, and therapists will have strong and probably conflicting opinions.

In both cases, many of the possible interventions will require additional resources, often from different budgets which are likely to be overstretched already and to have many competing claims on them. Others are simply a question of time, communication, and interdisciplinary working to improve the integration of care. In some cases, a small investment now might potentially mean less expenditure in the future. Needs assessment is one of the tools used to ensure that the health service uses its resources to improve the health of the population in the most efficient and effective way. The question of how best to employ limited resources, and the political and ethical debate about rationing of health care, is beyond the scope of this book. It is important to recognize, however, that needs assessment starts from the perspective of the population and its health status rather than from the perspective of the balance sheet, and that it does not shy away from identifying needs which may be difficult or expensive to meet—but nor does it shy away from identifying existing services which, for one reason or another, do not meet local need and may be inappropriate or superfluous.

Need, supply, and demand

We have assumed so far that the concept of 'health needs' is conceptually simple and readily understood, and that needs are easily identifiable in practice. Alas, this is not the case, and as with other apparently straightforward terms encountered in this book it is important to be clear about definition and meaning. Several different kinds of health needs can be identified:

- *felt needs* are an individual's (or community's) subjective perception of poor health, which may or may not be articulated

- *expressed needs* are felt needs which have been articulated by individuals (or communities), usually in order to seek help to overcome their perceived poor health

- *normative needs* are those defined in relation to an objective norm of health, often by a professional who identifies interventions appropriate for the expressed need

- *comparative need* reflects a judgement about how one set of (individual or community) needs measures up to another, for example on the basis of severity, extent, and the range of interventions available or provided.

Simple examples are set out in Table 6.2.

There is also a distinction to be made between *health* needs and *health care* needs—essentially a need for health as opposed to a need for health care. Examples of health needs could include 'growing pains', neglect, or anything else which compromises a child's well-being but may not be 'treatable' by health services, whereas health care needs are specific health problems, such as a fracture or bacterial infection, which can benefit from health services. Some health needs may, however, be met by providing services, but they may also require or benefit from action on a wider scale to tackle determinants of health such as poverty, pollution, nutrition, housing, transport policy, employment opportunities, income inequality, or social capital.

Needs can be classified as *felt, expressed, normative*, or *comparative*—and can also be divided into *health care needs* and *health needs*. Health care needs are met by health services, whereas health needs may benefit from wider social, environmental, and economic action.

Table 6.2 Examples of different types of needs

Type of need	Individual patient examples	Community example
Felt	A child with abdominal pain which he or she is aware of but does not complain of	Members of a community who are concerned about the speed of traffic in their road
Expressed	A child with abdominal pain which he or she has reported and sought help from a health care professional	A community which has voiced its concern about traffic safety to the local council
Normative	A child with abdominal pain which has been deemed to require treatment or further investigation	A community whose road is recognized by the council to need traffic calming after accident statistics and traffic use have been examined
Comparative	A child whose abdominal pain has been assessed by a health care professional as more serious than the conditions of others waiting (e.g. in A&E)	A community whose road has been judged a priority for installation of speed bumps after comparison of local data with other potential sites

In reality, the distinction between the two is sometimes not so clear-cut. Both health needs and health care needs can be influenced by socio-economic status, the physical and social environment, and cultural and religious beliefs. Some health care needs would disappear if wider social and environmental action was taken; and in the absence of such wider action, some health needs can be mitigated by providing health care services. Does the rising tide of childhood obesity, for example, represent a health need or a health care need? What about deteriorating asthma in a child living in damp and mouldy accommodation? Is it appropriate to consider anaemia in a late-weaned baby as a health care need?

Another categorization which is helpful in needs assessment is the triad of need, supply, and demand, which is often illustrated diagrammatically by three overlapping circles, as in Fig. 6.1.

Here, *need* (usually assumed here to be a normative, objectively defined need for health care) is compared to the population's *demand* for health care (not dissimilar to expressed need in the set of definitions above) and to the health care which is currently provided or *supplied*. Certain conditions or interventions may fall into one, two, or three of the circles. For example, antibiotic treatment for acute ear infections may be demanded and supplied, but may not be needed since most cases will resolve without it. Similarly, child protection services for abused children may be needed and supplied but not demanded; appropriate adolescent health services may be needed and demanded but not supplied. Neonatal intensive care falls into the centre of the diagram where all three categories overlap, but a vaccination programme for an eradicated disease falls outside it altogether since it is neither needed, supplied, nor demanded.

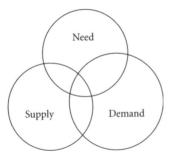

Fig. 6.1 The interrelated triad of need, supply, and demand.

Some authors impose a further qualification on needs which it is worth examining explicitly at this stage: that is, that health *care* needs exist only if an effective treatment is available for the condition in question. It follows that needs may change as research uncovers more therapies, or indeed exposes the ineffectiveness of established therapies. Thus a child with enlarged tonsils and troublesome but relatively infrequent tonsillitis would have been considered twenty years ago to have a need for tonsillectomy, but present wisdom suggests that, in the absence of complications such as sleep apnoea, he does not need any surgical intervention. (Sometimes practice in one country differs from that in another because of a different attitude to research on effectiveness or a different assessment of needs—for example, lead screening in children is regularly undertaken in the USA but not in the UK.) On the other hand, a child with a rare malignancy may be deemed to have no *health care* need in respect of active treatment, since no effective treatment has been identified for her condition, although she will have *health* needs for palliative care and support. However, that situation may change overnight with the publication of results from a research trial or a judgement by the National Institute for Clinical Effectiveness (NICE) that a new treatment merits general usage in the NHS.

Although it may seem logical to concentrate on those health care needs which we have the means to address, and to address with treatments of proven efficacy, it may also seem counterintuitive to define needs in such a conditional way. It is important to understand, however, how the niceties of definitions may affect policy decisions. Limiting health care needs to conditions for which interventions of proven efficacy exist may exclude conditions and therapies for which adequate research has not yet been conducted. If this is so, then it is vital to re-evaluate the situation regularly in the light of new information—and to ensure that needs assessment feeds into the research and development agenda by identifying key areas in which research is needed to guide the provision of health care.

This is a complex and potentially confusing area, and it may seem that detailed consideration of what constitutes a health or health care need is of limited value in terms of day-to-day practice. It is important, however, that those working in the field of child public health are aware of these issues and explore their own understanding, definitions, and value systems before venturing forth into the field.

Approaches to needs assessment

There are many approaches to health needs assessment, some of which are listed in the box below.

- Epidemiological
- Comparative
- Corporate
- Participatory
- Rapid appraisal

Needs assessment may focus on a particular condition (e.g. childhood diabetes), service (e.g. neonatal intensive care), or client group (e.g. children with learning difficulties), or it may be more open-ended, starting with a community and exploring its needs and problems to identify priority areas for more formal needs assessment.

Stevens and Raftery have described a tripartite framework for needs assessment which has been influential:

- **Epidemiological needs assessment** compares the demography and health status of the target population, the effectiveness of interventions for the problem(s) in question, and the local availability of services (see Fig. 6.2). It implicitly assumes, as described above, that needs only exist if effective remedies are available, and seeks to identify gaps in services for which there is a need. Epidemiological needs assessment requires the collection of a considerable amount of information if it is to be conducted properly: the availability of data from different sources is explored later in the chapter.

- **Comparative needs assessment** contrasts services available locally with those available to similar populations in other areas.

- **Corporate needs assessment** gathers the views, desires, and knowledge of a range of stakeholders with different perspectives and experience.

It is often useful to combine all three approaches—epidemiological, corporate, and comparative—in order to develop as full a picture as possible of the health status and health needs of the population in question. For example, consider a needs assessment for a local population of asylum seekers, focussing particularly on unaccompanied

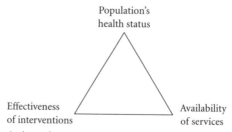

Fig. 6.2 Epidemiological needs assessment.

minors. *Epidemiological* information may be limited, but it would be important to find out as much as possible about the population (how many unaccompanied minors there were; their age, sex, and nationality; the main health problems affecting them), the current availability of services for them (e.g. the number registered with local GPs and any special provision such as a dedicated health visitor), and any evidence that could be found about effective means of providing health care for this group (e.g. models of care which had been piloted and evaluated elsewhere). The *comparative* approach would involve finding out what neighbouring districts had done or planned to do in order to meet the needs of a similar population. The *corporate* approach would mean seeking the views of these young people themselves, and those working with them (including health and social care professionals, and voluntary and community workers) as to how their health needs could most appropriately be met. Sometimes information from these different sources forms a coherent picture; sometimes conflicting priorities or views emerge which have to be explored and resolved. However, a combined approach generally provides a more comprehensive view and is more likely to yield appropriate solutions which meet with general agreement.

> **Epidemiological** needs assessment is based on information about the population's health status and the availability and effectiveness of health care. **Comparative** needs assessment assesses need and provision relative to other similar populations. **Corporate** needs assessment reflects the views of a range of stakeholders.

Other techniques have been developed which reflect these basic approaches but have their own particular characteristics which make them especially appropriate for certain situations. **Rapid appraisal** needs assessment suits our need for expeditious responses to the child public health agenda in the twenty-first century; and **participatory** needs assessment, which builds on the theme of community approaches to health promotion described in Chapter 4, focusses on the target community and helps it to appraise its own needs.

Rapid appraisal

Rapid appraisal aims to gather a variety of information and perspectives on local health and social needs swiftly, and to translate these findings equally swiftly into proposals for action. It is a technique which is particularly well suited to investigating the health needs of a well-defined neighbourhood or population, or in any situation where obtaining a speedy overview of the situation is more important than an exhaustive survey—an approach sometimes referred to in the trade as 'quick and dirty'. It can be used to provide a starting point for a local community development project or a more in-depth assessment of a specific issue or problem. Data are collected from three main sources:

- Interviews with a wide range of local informants
- Existing written records about the neighbourhood
- Observations made in the neighbourhood or in the homes of the interviewees.

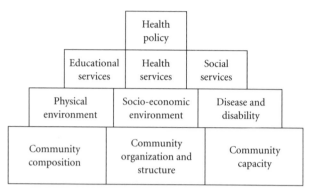

Fig. 6.3 Information pyramid for rapid appraisal. (Source: Murray, S. *BMJ* (1999) **318**:440–444, with permission from the BMJ Publishing Group.)

From these sources a 'pyramid' of data is assembled (see Fig. 6.3) describing the neighbourhood's problems and priorities. Data from one source are validated or rejected by checking with data from at least two other data sources or methods of data collection—a technique known as 'triangulation'. Informants are selected 'purposefully'—they are neither a comprehensive group nor a random sample, but have been identified by others as being in a good position to speak for the community on the issues involved. Professional views are often incorporated, as well as data collected from primary and secondary care.

Rapid appraisal needs assessment had its origins in work in developing countries, although it has subsequently been applied very effectively in the UK and other developed countries. An example of a suitable topic for rapid appraisal in child public health might exploring the needs of a rapidly-growing town with a burgeoning community of families with young children, where services (health, social care, education, transport) have not kept pace with population growth.

Participatory needs assessment

Participatory needs assessment also focusses early on action to address the issues raised, and puts the emphasis on needs assessment being done *by* rather than *to* a community. Its basic philosophy emphasizes the importance of encouraging communities to tackle for themselves the problems which they face and consider important. It is intimately related to the concept of community development and often aims to improve health through improving quality of life at a more general level for the community (see Fig. 6.4). The 'community' here, as in rapid appraisal needs assessment, may be people who live in the same area (such as an inner-city housing estate or remote rural community) or who have something else in common (for example, children with disabilities).

Health impact assessment

Health impact assessment is a related but different technique which is growing in importance as a public health tool. It has emerged from the more established process of environmental impact assessment, and is used to assess the likely impact on health

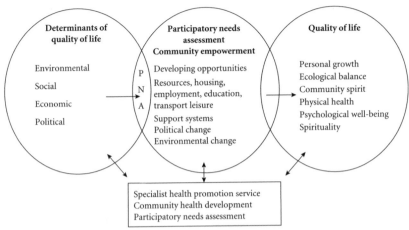

Fig. 6.4 The role of participatory needs assessment in improving quality of life. (Source: Public Health Medicine, London. Permission sought.)

of a planned development. It may be triggered by a community's concerns about, for example, a new traffic system or the closure of a mine, or may be part of the planning process for larger developments such as the construction of a bypass or a new airport runway. It typically takes a broad view, examining both the positive and negative, and direct and indirect health effects of the proposed scheme (including perhaps pollution, noise, accident risk, employment, social disruption) and looking at ways of minimizing or mitigating its impact. This may involve proposals to build a new playground or to redevelop an access road to take traffic away from a local village. Health impact assessment requires the gathering of qualitative and quantitative data, and incorporates both lay and expert perspectives, engaging the local community and a wide variety of professionals and interest groups.

Evidence and evaluation

We have already touched on the issues of effectiveness and evidence-based practice in public health during the discussion of health needs and community diagnosis. It is useful to explore a little further the usefulness, implications, and limitations of these concepts for public health practice. However, these are huge topics in their own right, and we do not propose to cover them in detail here: the further reading list at the end of the chapter includes references where the interested reader can find all they wish to know about evidence-based medicine and the design of randomized controlled trials and epidemiological studies (such as cohort and case-control studies) which are used to generate evidence of effectiveness.

The challenges of evidence-based practice in public health

As we saw in Chapter 3, the development of public health progammes in the past was often driven by belief and conviction, unsupported by research showing that the proposed interventions would be effective. While some of these interventions have been highly effective, others have failed or have been accompanied by unintended consequences. Developing an evidence base for public health is therefore important, but this is a more complicated business than developing an evidence base in clinical practice. For example, the complex interventions necessary to change behaviour are not well suited to randomized controlled trials, and it is rarely practical to trial changes in social policy. The World Health Organisation have recently announced that randomized controlled trials are 'unhelpful, inappropriate and unnecessarily expensive' in the evaluation of health promotion interventions. Many interventions (such as car seat belts and 'pedestrian friendly' fronts to cars to promote road safety, developed on the basis of engineering design calculations and tested in laboratory trials) have been introduced to great effect without controlled trials.

Some areas of public health practice pose particularly difficult problems. Due to the logistics and expense of the very long-term follow-up necessary, studies showing a direct impact of child health interventions on adult health are rare. There are, however, other approaches to evaluation which can and have been employed by those trying to establish the effectiveness of childhood interventions which might be expected to affect adult health. The evidence base in this area (described in Chapter 5) therefore relies on varying study methodologies and the findings from a range of studies.

There is a balance to be struck here between rigour and pragmatism—between the need to operate today within the realities of the messy everyday world where information, evidence, and certainty may all be lacking, and the ideal of a clear theoretical framework and strong evidence base on which to base public health action. It is important to remember that the lack of research evidence to guide clinical or public health interventions to meet certain individual or population health needs does not invalidate those needs nor mean that no attempt should be made to address them. Indeed, it is sometimes necessary to act without full information about effectiveness, either in the clinical or public health spheres—for example, in extreme cases where life is at risk or when something needs to be done for reasons of precaution, humanity, or commonsense.

The introduction of non-evidence-based policies continues today: UK governments have tried to improve children's diets in the past by providing free school milk and school meals to children whose families are on income support, and currently by providing fresh fruit to all school children, with the aim of improving growth and development and reducing adult disease risk. While these interventions seem like a good idea from a commonsense point of view, no studies have ever been undertaken to demonstrate that free provision would be followed by a sustained increase in consumption leading to better health outcomes.

> Developing an evidence base for public health is important, but is more complicated than in clinical practice. Randomized controlled trials may be neither feasible nor helpful. Many successful public health interventions have been introduced without prior evidence of effectiveness—but it is vital that such interventions are properly evaluated, so lessons can be learned for the future.

The importance of evaluation

Where interventions are introduced on the basis that it seems very likely that they will improve health rather than on the basis of unequivocal scientific evidence that this will happen, it is vital that they are properly evaluated in order that lessons can be learned about their effectiveness and operation, and future action can draw on the evidence yielded by past experience. Even in the case of evidence-based interventions, it is important that their implementation is monitored. Public health interventions are much more complex than clinical interventions, such as the administration of a drug, and much more can go wrong. Benefits demonstrated in well-funded research studies cannot always be replicated in practice, and research reports rarely provide the pragmatic details about the delivery of the intervention that can make the difference between success and failure.

> The critical assessment, on as objective basis as possible, of the degree to which entire services or their component parts...fulfil stated goals. (St Leger)

There is an extensive literature on health promotion evaluation, to which the 'Further reading' section again signposts those interested in this area, but a brief summary may be useful here. Health care evaluation has been defined as:

Cochrane first stressed the importance of evaluation and defined *effectiveness* and *efficiency* as key elements of performance to be assessed. Maxwell described six dimensions of quality which it is often helpful to consider when designing an evaluation: access, relevance, effectiveness, equity, acceptability, and efficiency. Holland has emphasized that acceptability can apply to professionals as well as the public.

Donabedian's influential model divides the system or intervention being studied into three elements to be examined during the evaluation:

* *Structure*: fixed resources and how they are organized
* *Process*: what is done (and how much); how activities and individuals interact
* *Outcome*: impact and end results

Evaluations of pilot or ongoing interventions may draw on the classical study designs, but as we have already seen these methods may be inappropriate and a more flexible approach may be needed. It is always important to include the perspective of users and the public; it is also vital to be clear what the intervention hopes to achieve, and to evaluate against specified targets and objectives wherever possible. In many cases, however, it is difficult or impractical to assess changes in the ultimate outcome—such as lower rates of premature death from coronary heart disease or cancer in the case of the school fruit scheme. Intermediate or proxy outcomes (such as changes in fruit consumption, population blood cholesterol levels, or childhood obesity) may have to be assessed, or it may be more appropriate to look at the process level in Donabedian's model (the number of children receiving free fruit in school as a result of the scheme being implemented).

Evaluating health promotion interventions presents a challenge. It is often necessary to look at intermediate outcomes rather than focussing on endpoints (e.g. mortality and morbidity), or to assess process measures or changes in knowledge, attitude, or behaviour.

Several authors have proposed ways of studying the effectiveness of health promotion interventions. Tannahill suggests examining their impact at several points on a hierarchy of change:

* Change in knowledge
* Change in attitude
* Change in behaviour
* Change in morbidity or mortality

Nutbeam suggests four levels for evaluation which build on Donabedian's model:

1 *Process*—unravelling the reasons for the success or failure of an intervention

2 *Impact*—evaluation against the programme's objectives, such as improved community participation or individual health literacy

3 *Intermediate outcomes*—the development of healthy lifestyles, healthy environments, or effective health services

4 *Health and social outcomes*—improvements in quality of life, reductions in morbidity, disability, or avoidable mortality

Some of the particular methodological challenges in developing an evidence base in public health include:

* Studies of interventions delivered through a school or community require very large, expensive trials in which the communities or schools are randomized to intervention and control group (cluster randomized controlled trials).

* Many public health interventions depend for their success on the implementation of several different approaches at the same time. Most trials aim to isolate the impact of individual approaches and these trials can miss synergistic or enabling effects.

* Public health interventions often depend on interpersonal skills which are not measured or reported in most trials. For example, the effectiveness of domiciliary health visiting is difficult to measure because of the multi-faceted nature of the interventions used by individual professionals and the fact that relationships and communication may count most in effecting change.

* Trials of public health interventions give priority to documenting the impact on health outcomes, and critical details about the process of implementation are often not gathered or reported. Such reports help practitioners know that something was or was not effective, but can leave doubts about what exactly the something was.

- Studies of interventions to promote health are limited by the lack of well-validated measures of well-being. Reliance on measures of disease or ill health is inappropriate in evaluating interventions which take a population approach, and 'ceiling' or 'floor' effects (when many participants score maximum at the beginning of the study) can mean that important improvements in health are missed.

Data sources

There are a number of sources of routinely collected data which can be used to build up a picture of the health needs of the population. These broadly divide into data which describes:

- populations (demographic data)
- health (often 'ill health') event data, such as mortality, hospital admissions, and consultations
- lifestyle and health status.

Below are shown some important routine sources of data on children and families in each category: some examples of data available from these sources were given in Chapter 1. Some useful data sources are listed at the end of this chapter.

Population data

Census data

Population censuses have been carried out in England and Wales since 1841, when the population was 15.9 million, with 46% aged under 20 and only 4% over the age of 65. They are carried out at ten-yearly intervals and provide key data for service planning and epidemiological studies. The population aged under 20 almost doubled between 1841 and 1911, from 7.3 million in 1841 to 14.4 million in 1911. Although the size of the overall population has continued to grow, the child population has actually fallen since this time, numbering 13.0 million (25.5% of the total) in 1991. Census data gives details of ethnic origin, occupation, and life-limiting illnesses.

Birth and death registration

Registration of births and deaths has been a statutory requirement in England and Wales since 1837. All births need to be registered by the parent within six weeks of delivery. There is no time limit after death for registration. Following registration of birth, a NHS number is provided which gives rights of access for the child to health services. NHS numbers are now generated at birth: this will be a useful advance for information systems, avoiding the difficulties which currently exist with duplicate or multiple records being generated as a result of name changes within the first few weeks of life. More efficient linkage of data on infants and mothers may improve care and research into early determinants of child morbidity.

Death registration data shows that life expectancy improved from 42 years to 75 years between 1841 and 1911. Currently there is a five-year gap in life expectancy

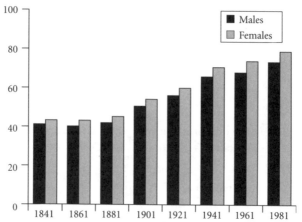

Fig. 6.5 Average life expectancy (years), 1841–1981 (Source: ONS).

between males and females, with females living longer. A gender difference in mortality exists throughout childhood and is reflected in differential morbidity patterns.

> Population data sources include the decennial census and birth and death registrations.

Health events

Information about illness and disability is less comprehensive than information about deaths. Data sources include hospital episode statistics and GP consultation data (Royal College of General Practitioners). These sources describe the common reasons why children and young people seek routine health care services (see Table 6.3). They are event-based rather than child-based, so they do not distinguish multiple events in a single child from single events in several children.

Hospital episode statistics (HES)

Hospital episode statistics (HES) contain the following information:

- Hospital name
- Health authority of residence
- Demographic details (NHS number, sex, birth date, postcode of usual address)
- Admission details (referring GP, admission/discharge details, method/source of admission)
- Consultant episode details (consultant code, specialty)
- Clinical diagnoses, operations, and procedures undertaken.

Table 6.3 Children consulting (rate per 10,000 children) by type of condition, 1991/2, England and Wales

Disease group	Age group (years)	
	0–4	5–15
All diseases and conditions	10 221	7234
Infectious and parasitic diseases	3648	1888
Neoplasms	54	88
Endocrine, nutritional, and metabolic disease, and immunity disorders	60	43
Disease of the blood and blood forming organs	58	56
Mental disorders	228	194
Diseases of the nervous system and sense organs	4252	1881
Diseases of the circulatory system	19	26
Diseases of the respiratory system	6471	3680
Diseases of the digestive system	834	306
Diseases of the genitourinary system	570	453
Complications of pregnancy, childbirth, and the puerperium	7	5
Diseases of the skin and subcutaneous tissue	2715	1418
Diseases of the musculoskeletal system and connective tissue	161	489
Congenital anomalies	217	59
Certain conditions originating in the perinatal period	173	0
Symptoms, signs, all ill-defined conditions	2721	1363
Injury and poisoning	1293	1375
Supplementary classification of factors influencing health status and contact with health services	5313	1140

(Source: *Morbidity statistics from general practice, 1991/2*)

Data is collected about all NHS hospital attendances and admissions; some GP consultation data is available too. Various coding systems are used to distinguish patients' conditions and any procedures carried out.

With the growth in community services and day cases, children are spending less time in hospital (Fig. 6.6). The number of out-patient consultations is increasing, but the data collected for out-patients is less comprehensive than that collected on in-patients (Fig. 6.7).

Most health care episode data is coded according to the health problem(s) triggering the event. Several different coding systems exist, the more common being the International Classification of Diseases (ICD), READ codes, SNOMED, and

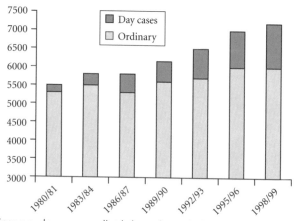

Fig. 6.6 Ordinary vs. day case paediatric in-patient admissions, 1980–99. (Source: ONS.)

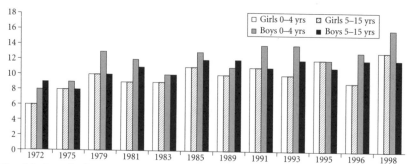

Fig. 6.7 Consultations in out-patients or casualty (% reporting attendance within a 3-month period). (Source: ONS Child Health Statistics, July 2000.)

Healthcare Resource Groups (HRGs). The ICD coding manual is constantly updated and is now in its tenth edition. It is the system used for coding hospital data. READ codes are used for general practice data.

Preventive care

Each UK area now has a computerized database of all children living in the area. This is used to manage preventive care services like immunization and surveillance episodes. It contains data about immunization and screening, together with some data on disability. The quality of data in these sytems is very variable and depends on investment both in software development and staff, together with the degree of interest taken by health professionals. Their usefulness for epidemiological studies varies from one area to another.

Chronic disease

Information about the incidence and prevalence of a small number of diseases—including congenital malformations, cancer, cerebral palsy, cystic fibrosis, and diabetes—is recorded in disease registers. Disease registers have four principal uses:

1. *Service planning* e.g. determining the numbers of children with severe communication disability who require special educational provision

2. *Epidemiological research* e.g. the evaluation of a prenatal screening programme (such as that for Down's syndrome) or geographical variation in congenital anomalies

3. *Clinical audit* e.g. using the register as a sampling frame to identify children with continence problems or challenging behaviour, for whom standards can be evaluated

4. *Individual patient care* e.g. to aid the co-ordination of multidisciplinary and inter-agency case reviews and planning meetings.

Some of the characteristics of a disease register are:

♦ it identifies individuals

♦ the individuals have certain characteristics in common

♦ it is longitudinal (a record kept over a period of time) and in some cases is systematically updated

♦ it records individuals within a geographically defined population.

The usefulness of a register can be compromised by poor initial planning, conflicting priorities for its use, incomplete or inaccurate data (case ascertainment), difficulties in maintaining staff interest and continuing managerial commitment, and failure to safeguard confidentiality and access arrangements.

Other sources of information on health and health care include child health databases (covering all children in an area) and disease registers for children with conditions such as cancer and diabetes.

Population-based survey data

General Household Survery

The General Household Survey commenced in 1971 and is a continuous survey of approximately 12,000 representative private households in Great Britain. Interviews are conducted with the adults in the household; a limited number of questions are included about children under the age of 16 years living in the household. A number of government departments use the data, which includes questions on housing, economic activity, pensions, leisure activities, education, and the family.

The health aspects covered include acute illness in the past two weeks, health during the previous year, the presence of chronic illness, consultations with a doctor, out-patient and in-patient visits to hospital, wearing of glasses or contact lenses, as well as smoking and drinking habits. Chronic illness affects one in five children aged 5–15, but only 50% report that their illness limits their day-to-day activities. Respiratory disease is the most common illness, reported by 7% of child respondents. This data is consistent with routine data showing the high prevalence of respiratory disorders in the child population.

Lifestyle and risk factors

There are a small number of other surveys which collect data on the prevalence of other specific illnesses, disabilities, health related lifestyles, and risk factors for ill health. In recent years national surveys have been carried out on the prevalence of disability and of mental illness in UK children. The WHO carries out an international survey on health behaviour of school children (HBSC) which includes data from the UK and allows international comparisons of trends in lifestyle factors (see Chapter 1).

Use of such data can help inform health promotion policy at several levels, from local (e.g. within a school) to national. The Schools Health Education Unit in Exeter also carries out surveys of health and health-related lifestyles in schools, providing data which help schools plan health promotion activities. As a very large number of schools have participated, the dataset is now large enough to be used to discern trends over recent years.

> Surveys can gather information on acute and chronic illness, disability, health-related lifestyles, and risk factors for ill health, from a sample of the population or a particular group such as a school. Surveys may be regular or ad hoc, local, national, or international.

Limitations of routine data for health needs assessment

Routine sources of data provide only a limited perspective on children's health. Increasingly, interest is being shown in measuring health needs from the perspective of children, young people, and their parents. There is a need to collect data on such indicators as health-related quality of life, functional health status, health-related educational capability, and family functioning.

Several groups in the USA, the UK and the European Union, and Australia are attempting to enhance routine data collection so that these aspects of health can be measured more accurately and universally. However, as the Medical Officer of Health for Nottingham noted in his Annual Report over 50 years ago:

> the collection of reliable information regarding the ills—both minor and grave—to which man is subject is a very slow process.

(W. Dodd, 1950)

> Data sources vary in terms of completeness and accuracy; their usefulness depends on many factors including the quality, appropriateness, and accessibility of their information, and commitment to their development and use.

Further reading

Evaluation

Cochrane, A. (1971). Effectiveness and efficiency: random reflections on health services. The 1971 Rock Carling Fellowship monograph. Nuffield Provincial Hospitals Trust.

Donabedian, A. (1988). The quality of care: how can it be assessed? *JAMA*; **260**(12):1743–8.

Holland, W.H. (ed.) (1983). *Evaluation of health care.* Oxford University Press, Oxford.

Maxwell, R.J. (1984). Perspectives in NHS management: quality assessment in health. *BMJ*; **288**: 1470–2.

St Leger, A.S., Schnieden, H., and Walsworth–Bell, J.P. (1992). *Evaluating health services' effectiveness: a guide for health professionals, service managers and policy makers.* Open University Press, Buckingham.

Needs assessment and community diagnosis

Stevens, A. and Gillam, S. (1998). Needs assessment: from theory to practice. *BMJ*; **316**:1448–52.

Stevens, A. and Raftery, J. (1994). *Healthcare needs assessment: the epidemiologically based needs assessment reviews.* Radcliffe Medical Press, Oxford.

Cook, J., Pechevis, M., and Waterston, T. (1995). Community diagnosis and participation. In *European Textbook of Social Paediatrics* (B. Lindstrom and N. Spencer (eds.)). Oxford University Press, Oxford.

Evidence-based medicine

Nutbeam, D. (1999). Making the case for health promotion: the questions to be answered. In *The evidence of health promotion effectiveness: shaping public health in a new Europe* (D. Boddy, ed.). EU Brussels.

Sackett, D.L., Scott Richardson, W., Rosenberg, W., and Brian Haynes, R. (1997). *Evidence based medicine.* Churchill Livingstone.

Thorogood, M. and Coombes, Y. (1999). *Evaluating health promotion: Practice and Methods.* Oxford University Press, Oxford.

Registers

Abra, A. and Woodroffe, C. (1991). A special conditions register. *Archives of Disease in Childhood*; **66**:927–30.

Blair, M.E. and Hutchison, T. (1997). Special needs registers—dreams and nightmares. In *Progress in community child health 2*, (ed. Spencer, N.), pp. 57–67. Churchill Livingstone.

Sources of data on child health

Botting, B. (ed.) *The health of our children decennial supplement.* Office for National Statistics (ONS), London.

ONS website: *www.ons.gov.uk.*

Woodroffe, C., Glickman, M., Barker, M., and Power, C. (1993). *Children, teenagers and health—the key data.* Open University, Buckingham.

Chapter 7

Using child public health techniques—some practical examples

In this chapter we give a number of practical worked examples relating to key areas of child public health for health professionals and their colleagues. The first describes the general process, for a newly appointed community paediatrician, of making a community diagnosis; the rest address specific problems. For each, a case scenario is described and there is a short review of the epidemiology, a list of the stakeholders likely to be involved, a survey of the evidence, and a suggested practical approach to tackling the problem. The framework for action is based on the concepts and information presented in earlier chapters.

Scenario A

Karen 'walks the patch'

This example describes the route taken by a community paediatrician taking up a new post in a deprived area of a large city, and wishing to assess the health and social needs of the local child population with the help of local primary care teams and public health specialists. Health visitors and other professionals with a geographical base use the phrase 'walking the patch' to describe what they do when coming into post for the first time and getting to know their case load. The term reflects the fact that the local community is the locus of interaction (as opposed to a GP's case load, for example, which might span several different distinct communities). Similarly, a new community paediatrician will often be allocated a 'patch' or geographical locality within which to base their activities.

Case study

Karen Blackford has been appointed as a paediatrician with an interest in public health in a former mill town in the North of England called Milton. It is well known for its high unemployment rate and relatively large child population. There have been a number of high-profile cases in the area including two child deaths from abuse in the past three years and an outbreak of measles for the first time in 20 years. Children and young people who misuse drugs are over-represented compared to the norms for the region, and vandalism and car crime is high.

Karen decides that she would like to take a systematic approach to finding out about the child health problems in the area and convenes a meeting with a range of local professionals to discuss this project. Those attending include representatives from local primary care teams, the public health lead for children within Milton's primary care organization (e.g. PCT in England), and the designated nurse for child protection. They agree that there has been little emphasis on child health locally, and that few recent initiatives have addressed children's needs. This is partly due to competing national targets and priorities in adult health which have preoccupied service planners, and partly to the lack of a clear and united voice advocating for children in Milton. Karen suggests that a more co-ordinated approach should begin with a needs assessment.

Discussion at the meeting is recorded on flip charts and is later typed up and circulated to participants as a series of agreed actions and points to consider. The notes read as follows:

- Public health department to obtain available child health data.
- Need list of key people delivering services in the patch for Karen to meet: informants to be identified by GPs, community nurses, and local community development officer.
- Need to include other agencies—social services, education, police, youth offending team, voluntary sector, community leaders.
- Need to map current provision and possibilities (e.g. potential for community development work in Beechlands housing estate—family centre there run by National Children's Home).
- Community-based mental health services for children a particular problem.
- Any new interventions must meet needs identified by local community, must be sustainable, and must be evaluated.

Further discussion with the public health lead for children's services helps Karen to frame her approach in terms of a formal needs assessment, combining elements of both corporate and epidemiological approaches and of community participation (as described in Chapter 6). They set out the following framework:

Corporate needs assessment
- Stakeholder views—including young people and families, professionals from different agencies and voluntary sector—about key health problems and interventions needed.

Epidemiological needs assessment
- Routine and other data on demography, morbidity, mortality of local child population.
- Information on current local services—health, social care, voluntary sector.
- Evidence of effectiveness, especially in relation to possible new services or developments.

Community participation
- Encourage wide range of local people to be involved in identifying problems and suggesting solutions.
- Be prepared to support local community in developing its own initiatives.

Child health data from routine data sources/local surveys

The data presented to Karen by the public health department are somewhat limited. Although there is good data on mortality, information on morbidity is sparse and is suspected to be unreliable and incomplete. Karen is particularly interested in information about child accidents and behavioural problems which are not available from routine sources. The data available is illustrated in Table 7.1.

Local health visiting and school nursing 'profile' data helps to fill in some of the gaps, and useful information is also obtained from other sources. The social services department is able to provide detailed data on looked after children from its 'Quality Protects' returns and on children on the child protection register. The youth offending team has information on young people's involvement in crime; and the education department provides details of school exclusions, truancy, and attendance at special schools, including those for children with emotional and behavioural difficulties. The police have data on road traffic accidents involving children. Some GP practices which have been involved in a pilot project to promote recording and accessibility of information on their computer system are able to provide details of consultations and referrals for patients under 16. Karen also accesses online data on neighbourhood statistics to help build up a profile of the local area, especially in relation to deprivation. The Index of Multiple Deprivation scores for the four wards in Milton place them between the 3000th and 7000th most deprived wards out of 8414 in England and Wales, and the Child Poverty Index scores tell a similar story.

Table 7.1 Child health data from routine sources

Size and breakdown of child population under 15s	49,500
Births	3400 births per year
Proportion birth weight below 2.5 kg	7.4%
Neonatal mortality rate	6 in 1000
Infant mortality rate	7.3 in 1000
Breast-feeding rate at birth	55%
Coverage of six-week check	95%
Child mortality and causes of death	20 per yr.—mainly prematurity, accidents, cancer, infection, and one case of NAI in the last year
Teenage pregnancies	63 in 1000 women aged 14–19
Hospital out-patient consultation/A&E attendance	16% (varies from 3%–34% depending on local authority ward deprivation indices)
Immunization rate (completion of primary course)	87%
Immunization rate (MMR)	85%

Lack of appropriate health data is a common problem, and one of the tasks of a public health oriented paediatrician is to identify information that is needed, what is available routinely, and what must be collected specifically. It is increasingly important for all health professionals to become familiar with child health information systems and data collection so as to inform their future development and improvement.

Discussion with key health professionals and local people

Over the course of several weeks Karen meets a wide variety of people from the health sector, the local authority, and local voluntary organizations. They are listed in the box below.

Stakeholders in child health in West Milton

Health visitor representative on primary care organization (PCT) board
Chief Executive of primary care organization (PCT)
Lead school nurse
Senior social worker for children's services
Senior educational psychologist
Psychologist from child and mental health service
Other community paediatricians
Head of NCH family centre
Parents who attend the family centre
Local councillor
Youth workers
Educational social workers
Heads of local schools

Karen wanted to meet children and young people to find out what they think about local services and what they perceive as the key health and social problems they face. She is told of a study that has recently been completed by school nurses in the area, involving a series of workshops facilitated by a youth worker, to ascertain the views of children and young people on health issues. Karen is able to attend a follow-up focus group meeting at which some of the findings are discussed.

Some of the information provided by stakeholders is described below.

Health visitor Health visitors are trained to collect information on populations and have developed expertise in community profiling, making them an important resource in community diagnosis. Mandy covers one of the most deprived estates in the patch (Beechlands). The information she has obtained through community profiling enables her to identify the main problems in children's health locally, the strengths of the community, and which families are particularly high-risk. She considers that the main problems are in child behaviour and nutrition, accidents, and delayed speech and language development.

School nurse Liz is the school nurse for the largest of the local secondary schools. She has to cover several other schools and is conscious that she has insufficient time to meet the needs of the pupils adequately. She is aware that stress levels are high among young people and that there are many unresolved emotional and behavioural problems. A recent survey of behaviour and attitudes in local schools revealed much high-risk behaviour especially in relation to sexual health and drug and alcohol misuse.

GP Rajiv is a partner in a five-doctor practice that covers the same estate as Mandy. He is conscious of a poor understanding of health and disease among his patients and feels that local health services are not always appropriately used. There are many call-outs at night for minor complaints such as raised temperature, upper respiratory infection, or crying in a baby. He reports a high level of smoking locally, examples of inadequate care of young children, excessive use of junk foods, and high rates of teenage pregnancy.

Parents The parents attending the family centre describe a different set of problems, including difficulty in getting appointments to see the doctor, difficulty in understanding what the doctors say, lack of local play facilities for children, poor public transport, and fear of letting children play outside because of 'problem families' in the neighbourhood.

Children and young people Stress, community safety, and concerns about the environment are all important issues for young people locally. Lack of job prospects, conflict with parents and teachers, and a failure to have their point of view taken into account exacerbate the situation for them. They don't feel local health services are accessible or appropriate to their needs and are reluctant to go and see the local GP about 'private health problems'.

Social worker Mavis has worked in Milton for ten years and is despondent about the impact of budget cuts and difficulties in recruiting new staff which have put increasing pressure on her team. She feels the needs of families and children are increasing all the time and that there is less scope to intervene except in the most serious cases, so that problems often get out of hand before they can be addressed. She is particularly worried about the parenting skills of very young mothers and the difficulty in providing adequate support to care leavers.

Chief Executive of primary care organization Although sympathetic to the needs of children in Milton, Sean's main concern is to bring the PCT into financial balance and to meet the many 'must-do' targets the government has set for the next few years—few of which concern children. He is keen to support initiatives mentioned in the NHS Plan such as 'Sure Start', universal neonatal hearing screening, breast-feeding, and parenting programmes, and to ensure that community staff employed by the PCT are working effectively.

Karen also maps existing services, including the current work of the child health team in her patch (including health visitors and school and community nurses) and considers their suggestions about reprioritization. It is agreed that this will be discussed collectively at a later stage in the light of the needs assessment findings and evidence base. The public health lead searches the literature for evidence of effectiveness in relation to certain interventions which have been proposed.

A follow-up meeting is convened to present and discuss findings from the needs assessment process. Despite differences in perspective, clear priorities for child health emerge from the discussions with local stakeholders. These include a focus on children in different age groups: preschool children, younger school-age children, and teenagers.

Milton community diagnosis—key problems in child health

All children: poverty and inequalities in health, community safety, parenting education and support, mental health
Preschool children: behaviour problems, delayed development, poor nutrition, low coverage of immunizations, availability of child care and nursery provision
Primary school children: accidents, nutrition, dental health
Teenagers: nutrition, high-risk behaviour (drugs, alcohol, sexual health, accidents)

Next steps

It is clear that the 'community diagnosis' requires an inter-agency approach over a long period of time, a re-evaluation of current services and work practices, and a clarity about the evidence base for improvement. Karen is conscious of the fact that, whilst there is no time like the present for assessing problems and scoping possible solutions, as a newcomer to the area she needs to tread carefully at first in terms of action. It will be essential for her to spend time building the relationships which will be vital to sustained success in tackling the problems identified and to get a better understanding of 'how things work' locally. A measured and appropriate response is likely to be more effective than an attempt to solve every problem at once.

Together with the primary care and public health leads, an inter-agency child health improvement team is developed with a wide membership, under the aegis of the primary care organization's public health department. The team recognizes that concerted action and the involvement of local people and professionals working together will be vital, and that the first step is to agree priority areas to focus on initially. As well as the most pressing problems identified by local stakeholders, these might include a couple of projects identified as 'early winners' likely to yield fairly swift results, and areas in which national targets have been set or which can benefit from specific funding streams. The PCT may be able to find non-recurrent funding for some short-term projects.

It is agreed that three workshops will be held in different localities within the patch to discuss possible projects and developments. There will also be two workshops for children and young people, facilitated by experienced youth workers. The team agrees that the criteria for taking forward any new initiative in child health will be:

- Perceived importance in the eyes of local people
- Possible to monitor outcome

+ Some evidence of effectiveness of the proposed action and therefore likelihood of success

+ Sustainability

+ Tackles structural issues (e.g. not just provision of information)

+ Includes some element of parent empowerment

The workshops are successful and many specific areas for action are raised which reflect the concerns of local people, including play areas for children, nursery and child care provision, shopping facilities, and the negative impact of recent service cuts, especially in social services. It is agreed that councillors will take these concerns to the relevant local authority planning groups. The child health team also volunteer to take on an advocacy role in supporting parents such as the group which has already formed to lobby the transport and housing departments to improve road safety and ensure windows and railings are repaired on the local estate. The police representatives at the workshops agree to feed back community safety concerns and to discuss these further with local residents.

The topics of greatest importance for the community in relation to health service provision are children's behaviour problems, accident prevention, and adolescent health issues. The latter include access to services; drug, tobacco, and alcohol use; stress; sexual health issues; and relative lack of physical fitness. Proposals for action include:

+ a 'Sure Start' bid

+ developing a 'healthy living' centre in Beechlands

+ parenting programmes

+ starting a community-run nursery

+ a needle exchange designed to be accessible to young people

+ developing a 'BodyZone' scheme (outreach health information and advice centre) and breakfast club in local schools

+ 'Healthy Schools' projects

+ a loan scheme for home safety equipment

+ funding of community worker to help with initiating specific local projects.

Several of these will require considerable development work, which the child health improvement team agrees to consider. Karen and the public health lead will explore the time-scale for Sure Start scheme bids. Other individuals are invited to submit brief proposals for smaller projects which might be started with the help of the PCT's short-term funding: these include the breakfast club, community nursery, and safety equipment loan scheme. Increasing awareness of alternative sources of out-of-hours health advice, such as NHS Direct, was also felt to be important, and Karen agrees to seek the help of her community team in promoting this.

In developing new initiatives, time-scale and sustainability are all-important. Change does not come quickly and it is depressing to find that funding has run out after two or three years just as the benefits of an intervention are becoming apparent. Before starting a new project, there needs to be agreement about how it will be continued within mainstream resources once any special funding has been used up.

The developments proposed in Milton are likely to be too extensive to introduce all at once: several involve many steps which will require careful consideration and planning, and of course the identification of funding, and each will need to be managed by someone who is able to take a global view of their aims. A phased development over a number of years is likely to be more effective and feasible. Appropriate public accountability is also vital to ensure a long-term commitment to sustaining change. However, the process of needs assessment has been successful in identifying some key problems and possible solutions, and has also been of benefit in developing relationships between different agencies, and between professionals and the community. Engaging local people and encouraging them to participate in the process has already helped to empower them and to tap into the considerable resources of the community. It will be important, however, not to raise unreasonable expectations and to ensure that momentum is sustained in order that disillusion does not follow.

In practice, public health projects often come in smaller and less comprehensive packages than this example suggests, so that the action needed is not quite so daunting. The remaining scenarios focus more closely on a number of specific problems and interventions.

Further reading

Alperstein, G. and Nossar, V. (1998). Key interventions for the health improvement of children and youth: a population based approach. *Ambulatory Child Health*; 4:295–306.

Children and Young People's Unit (2001). *Learning to listen: Core principles for the involvement of children and young people.* CYPU, London.

Cook, J., Pechevis, M., and Waterston, T. (1995). Community diagnosis and participation. In *European textbook of social paediatrics* (B. Lindstrom and N. Spencer, eds.). Oxford University Press, Oxford.

Eisenstadt, N. (2002). Sure start: Key principles and ethos. *Child care, health and development*; 28:3–4.

Sure start website http://www.dfes.gov.uk/sure start

Waterston, T. (1995). How can child health services contribute to a reduction in health inequalities in childhood? In *Progress in community child health* (N. Spencer, ed.), pp. 11–29. Churchill Livingstone.

Scenario B

Prevention of behaviour problems and the promotion of mental health

Case study

Sue Bailey, a health visitor attached to Burnwood Surgery, has a large case-load and is concerned that she is not able to give enough support to families who are experiencing problems with their children's behaviour. She has the feeling that the number of pre-school and reception class children with conduct problems is growing, and that the families she is visiting feel powerless to do anything about the problem. The waiting list for assessment at the local child and adolescent mental health service is now 15 months, and the child psychiatrists are advising that they can only see children who are in trouble with the police or at risk of being taken into care. She has discussed her impressions with the leader of Burnwood's preschool (playgroup), the Bright Stars Nursery, and the school nurse at Pinforth Primary School. These all agree that there is a problem and that the problem is growing. Sue brings her concerns to a primary care team meeting.

Background epidemiology

Emotional and behavioural problems are common. At the severe end of the scale they are classified into conduct disorder, oppositional defiancy disorder, attention deficit hyperactivity disorder (ADHD), phobias, and depression. However, all the symptoms and behaviours which characterize these mental health problems are exhibited by normal children from time to time, so it is the frequency and constellation of behaviour and symptoms which determine the diagnosis. The prevalence of these problems therefore depends on the diagnostic criteria used, which change from time to time.

As described in Chapter 2, recent UK surveys suggest that the prevalence of psychiatrically abnormal behaviour is around 10% of 5–11 year olds, and that it may be as high as 20% in urban areas. Because diagnostic criteria and methods of measurement vary, precise trends over time are difficult to determine, but a number of studies support the view of professionals working with children that such problems are becoming more common. A recent national survey of childhood disability identified behaviour problems as the single most important cause of functional disability in childhood. Behaviour problems blight children's lives, making it difficult for them to learn at school and to make friends with their peers. As Chapter 5 makes clear, most children do not grow out of these problems. As adolescents they are at high risk of school failure, delinquency, substance misuse, teenage pregnancy, violence, and crime. As adults they are at high risk of personality disorder, depression, anxiety, drug and alcohol abuse, and marital breakdown.

Studies on the aetiology of behaviour problems suggest that both genetic and environmental factors are involved. The environmental factors are both social and psychological. Behaviour problems are more common amongst families living in poverty, in the children of teenage parents, and children of parents with mental illness. However, because of the relatively small number of children living in these circumstances, the majority of children with behaviour problems do not have these predisposing factors (see Chapter 4, p.141). There is some evidence to suggest that behaviour problems may be caused or exacerbated by sensitivity to chemicals in food and drinks. They are also much more common in families which show little affection to their children, criticize them frequently and praise them rarely, take little interest in what they are doing at school or elsewhere, have inconsistent rules and boundaries, and mete out harsh discipline. They are uncommon in families where parents enjoy their children, accept them for being rather than doing, show interest in what they are doing, encourage them to try new things, support the development of autonomy, have clear boundaries for unacceptable behaviour, and enforce these boundaries with positive discipline.

What works?

Intervention studies have concentrated on two areas—programmes for parents and programmes for children (both preschool and at school). Redistribution of income and elimination of child poverty would be very likely to reduce these problems, but could not eliminate them. There have not been any studies of the effect of redistributive interventions on childhood behaviour problems. There are no high quality randomized controlled trials of dietary interventions, but many parents have observed that their children benefit from the elimination of food colourings, caffeine, and other additives from their diet.

Community interventions to date have taken one of three approaches: secondary prevention or treatment for families with established behaviour problems; primary prevention targeted at families in high-risk areas; and primary prevention taking a universal or population approach (see Chapter 4). Home visiting programmes targeted at high-risk families are effective in the first year of life and a range of different programmes have been tested. All include some element of support for the parent and all depend on the visitor being able to establish an empathetic, respectful relationship with parents. They aim to empower parents and to support the development of their mental health. The programmes may aim to help parents become more receptive and attuned to their babies' needs, promoting attachment. They may teach cognitive behavioural approaches to mothers suffering depression. They may teach child development, baby massage, behaviour management and diet; and they may encourage uptake of preventive services.

Group-based parenting programmes are effective with parents of 3–8 year olds, both as secondary and primary prevention, and trials with under fours are promising. They also have a beneficial impact on mothers' mental health. There are different types of programmes, but most run for 10–12 weeks, meeting for 2 hours a week, involving 8–12 parents (potentially of both sexes, but mothers are more likely to come). They use video, role modelling, and homework.

Behaviourist programmes help parents learn to let their children take the lead when they play with them and teach positive discipline techniques (rewarding good behaviour and ignoring bad, establishing clear boundaries, and using time out or withdrawal of privileges, rather than physical punishment or shouting). The relationship programmes also teach positive discipline but aim as well to help parents identify the emotional distress lying behind difficult behaviour and to address that, at the same time as establishing and maintaining clear boundaries. They also help parents understand their own emotional distress and problem behaviours and the contribution they may be making to the problem. They increase parents' sensitivity and respect for their children—skills which are essential to authoritative parenting. Programmes may also help parents share songs, books, and stories with their children. The effectiveness of such programmes seems to depend as much on the skills of the group leaders as on the programme itself. Group leaders need to be trained in facilitation skills as well as in the programme's approach.

Preschool and day nursery programmes often run alongside early parenting interventions. They take babies and young children from deprived families for up to five days a week, aiming to give children a positive start from an educational point of view and to support the development of social skills. Head Start in the USA is an example of such a programme.

School-based programmes may focus on primary or secondary prevention. They may aim to teach social competence, anger management, violence prevention, and/or emotional literacy to children. They may be offered, in special groups or classes, to children whom teachers have identified as being at risk, or they may be offered to all children. The programmes which are most successful are those which take a whole-school approach, involving all staff as well as all pupils, and which are carried out over a long time.

A range of other approaches to supporting parents have also been shown to be valuable, both on their own and as an adjunct to the programmes decribed above. They include drop-in centres which may be run by parents or professionals. These offer mutual support and advice and sometimes a range of programmes to parents. They also include volunteer home visiting schemes such as Home Start and Community Mothers, together with books, videos, and television programmes—all of which help to normalize and destigmatize parenting programmes.

Who are the stakeholders?

All the statutory agencies, including health, education, social services, probation, police, and criminal justice have an interest in preventing behaviour problems and their sequelae. Communities and local business can also suffer the consequences of petty crime and violence. Parents find childhood behaviour problems very distressing, as do other children in the same classroom or school. The number and range of stakeholders is therefore large.

An approach

The first time Sue tried to raise the problem at a primary care team meeting she was unable to promote any interest. The team were concerned with the establishment of their primary care trust and had explicitly agreed that health promotion was to take a back seat. Frustrated, Sue discussed the problem with Pinforth school nurse and six months later they tried again. This time the team agreed to set up a meeting with the social work manager and the head teacher of Pinforth. The midwife and practice manager were also invited. Sue managed to find a systematic review of parenting interventions to take to the meeting and invited a colleague from a neighbouring health district who had experience of running groups to attend. A chance discussion with a parent in a clinic made Sue aware that the Catholic Church in Burnswood had run a parenting programme a year ago. After discussion with the team she also invited the priest to the meeting.

At the meeting there was a lot of debate about the extent to which behaviour problems were due to genes, to deprivation, or to parenting. Several people were very sceptical about whether parents could change. The possibility of screening for behaviour problems was discussed and rejected because it had been shown not to work. The priest was able to describe what some of his parishioners had said to him about their programme and the impact it had had on their lives. The health visitor from the neighbouring district backed him up, saying that the parents in her group had felt supported and empowered. She did, however, point out that it was quite difficult to get parents to come. Most were already very over-committed and some were suspicious that they might labelled as bad parents. She also said that some of her parents had said the groups weren't long enough and that they wanted more. Sue was able to produce the evidence of effectiveness and to explain that parenting interventions need to tread a very careful line between victim blaming and support. She said she liked the idea of universal programmes because they were not stigmatizing and because she had looked at one of them and realised that there were ideas in the programme she did not know about and would like to try herself.

Funding and possible venues for programmes were discussed. All agreed that social services' premises were not suitable, but that the school, the church hall, and the surgery were possibilities. It was agreed that the church would try to set up another group and Sue would attend as a parent. She would also be released for three days training in running a parenting programme and would try and find a colleague who was interested in co-leading. When she had been trained, the practice would start to invite parents of rising threes to attend a group, and the practice health visitors and teachers would make sure that parents of children with troubling behaviour were encouraged to attend. When enough parents (probably 15, to allow for drop-outs) had agreed to come, Sue would run a group at four o'clock in the school, with an after-school club/crèche for those who needed it. The practice manager suggested that funding for the extra health visitor hours could come from the small budget the practice had earmarked for health promotion in their health improvement plan. Social services agreed to fund the crèche using money from an 'innovations fund'.

The team agreed to meet again when the midwife had had a chance to find out about antenatal and post-natal programmes and the head teacher had followed up something she had heard at a head teachers' meeting last year about a home–school linked mental health programme. She thought she might be able to get funding for this from the County Council's citizenship education fund. The priest said he would investigate the possibility of charitable donations from local businesses. The social work manager agreed to approach the police and probation service to see whether they would contribute to funding. All agreed that they would need to keep reviewing the situation and that they were unlikely to see any dramatic changes in mental health for some time.

Further reading

Barlow, J. and Stewart–Brown, S. (2001). Behaviour problems and parent education programs. *Developmental and Behavioral Pediatrics*, **21**:356–70.

Barlow, J., Coren, E., Stewart–Brown, S. (2002). Meta-analysis of the effectiveness of parenting programmes in improving maternal psychosocial health. *British Journal of General Practice*, **52**:223–33.

Barnes, J. (2002). *From pregnancy to early childhood: early interventions to enhance the mental health of children and families.* Mental Health Foundation, London. Available on the Mental Health Foundation website: *www.mentalhealth.org.uk*

Committee on Integrating the Science of Early Childhood Development (2000). Promoting healthy development through interventions. In *From neurons to neighborhoods: the science of early childhood development.* National Academy Press, Washington DC.

Erickson, M.F., Korfmacher, J., and Egeland, B. Attachments past and present: implications for therapeutic intervention with mother infant dyads. In *Development and psychopathology*. Cambridge University Press, New York.

MacLeod, J. and Nelson, G. (2000). Programmes for the promotion of family wellness and the prevention of child maltreatment: a meta-analytic review. *Child Abuse and Neglect*, **24**:1127–49.

Marshall, J. and Watt, P. (1999). *Child behaviour problems: a literature review of its size, nature and prevention interventions*. The Interagency Committee on Children's Futures, 189 Royal Street East, Perth, Western Australia.

Weare, K. (2000). *Promoting mental, emotional and social health: a whole school approach*. Routledge, London.

Scenario C
Reduction of teenage pregnancy and sexually transmitted infections through school-based approaches

Case study

Blatchworth Secondary School is in the local newspaper again because a third school-aged pregnancy has occurred in a single term. At the same time, the school nurses in the surrounding primary schools have been approached by teachers about the increasing demands for appropriate sanitary facilities for menstruating girls. These two issues are raised at a local governors' meeting and advice is sought from the local health community.

Background epidemiology

As we saw in Chapter 1 (Fig. 1.24), the UK has the highest level of teenage pregnancy in Europe and one of the highest in the world. In addition, the rate of sexually transmitted infection is rising, particularly chlamydia and HIV in heterosexuals. The age at which girls reach menarche is coming down. A greater proportion of girls are menstruating in primary school, resulting in the need for better provision of sanitary support within the school setting. These two areas of sexual health have converged and raised wider issues about the process and timing of sex education amongst school children.

Why does the UK have such a high rate of teenage pregnancy? A number of possible reasons are cited, among them the well-recognized antipathy on the part of parents (and school governors) towards discussion of sex and the puritan attitudes to sex education in schools. This is a controversial area to tackle, as there is still opposition to sex education from those who believe, wrongly, that more education will lead to more sex. There is disquiet (and disapproval by adults) over attitudes to sexual intercourse among the young, yet there are very widespread images in the media of sexuality in quite young children, which research in the USA has shown to influence attitudes. The media is hard to control and there is an intimate connection between media imagery and the marketing of clothes and cosmetics.

Teenage parents are known to be poorer, less well educated, and more likely to be unsupported emotionally and financially. The consequences for their children include a higher mortality rate in the perinatal period and infancy, increased use of medical services, and increased risk of child abuse and neglect. Some have argued that given sufficient support by social and education services, and the wider community, teenage parents and their children can be helped considerably. However, the costs to the state of teenage pregnancy are high, and there is great merit in preventing this mostly adverse event.

What works?

Sex education can be effective in changing practice, and peer education programmes are beneficial. However, the way that sex education is carried out is very important. It has been shown that young people need ready access to a clinical service where they can obtain advice and provision such as emergency contraception. It is important that such services are accepting and non-judgmental. A recent systematic review of teenage pregnancy prevention revealed that in countries where children and their carers are 'open' in their attitudes to sexual relationships, and are prepared to discuss these, the prevalence of pregnancy is lower.

Who are the stakeholders?

Children and young people, parents, teachers and school governors, obstetricians and gynaecologists, family planning doctors, paediatricians, the local education authority, and health promotion unit all have an interest.

An approach

Jeanine and Sarah, the school nurse and welfare assistant for Blatchworth, decide that it would be useful to present the issues to the various stakeholders. Together with the local health promotion unit (HPU), they develop a campaign involving local radio and TV coverage which aims to highlight the differences in teenage pregnancy rates in the city and the consequences of such pregnancies. Jeanine has a close relationship with the head of Year 6 in the school, and using information from the HPU they set up a competition to produce their own materials for peer teaching. These will cover family life, education, relationships, and parenting—rather than just sexual activities, contraception, and the prevention of sexually transmitted diseases. A local DJ from the radio station is invited to the school to give out the prize to the winner and highlight the issue on his next show.

To maintain momentum, Jeanine liaises closely with the teacher responsible for health matters in the school and ensures that the topic of sexual health is fully integrated into the personal, social, and health education (PSHE) curriculum at the school, and that the support of the governors is maintained. Blatchworth School decides to take a stance on the marketing of sex in the media, particularly that aimed at young people, by raising awareness amongst TV advertisers and producers of the evidence linking media exposure and sexual promiscuity in young people. The media were quick to pick up the story of the pregnant schoolgirls in the first place and are willing to run a story about how the school is responding. The editor of the local paper advises his advertising section, as a future policy, not to publish any more pictures which might be considered sexually promiscuous.

Dr Manson and Dr Burns (local paediatrician and family planning doctor) work closely with the school nurses and the district co-ordinator for teenage pregnancy reduction to set a standard for local availability of confidential drop-in contraceptive and sexual disease services in or near schools, where emergency contraception is also on offer. They present a business case to the Primary Care Trust which takes account of new national funding schemes for teenage pregnancy reduction, and establish a monitoring system which records clinical and drop-in consultation rates.

Environmental adaptations need to be considered in order to provide sanitary towel dispenser and disposal facilities in the primary schools. This is raised as an item to be taken into account during the schools' budget-setting process. The adaptations proposed are costed and included in the standard building specification for future schools planned by the education authority.

Jeanine and Sarah also invite two ex-pupils who have had babies in the past two years to give a talk to the classes currently in their final year at school. The focus is on the real hardships experienced (such as loss of their childhood and teenage years, new responsibilities, lack of finance or short-term further education opportunities) as well as the positive aspects of early motherhood. They conclude with a message to their younger peers to try and find employment and other occupational opportunities and avoid pregnancy as a 'way out' of an undesirable social situation.

What happened next?

The group met and concluded that they had done well so far, but that they might need to meet again in another year to review progress. Meanwhile, they would keep an eye on trends in teenage pregnancy rates and an ear to the group for information about how the services they had put in place were working.

Further reading

DiCenson, A., Guyatt, G., Willan, A., and Griffith, L. (2002). Interventions to reduce unintended pregnancies among adolescents: systematic review of randomized controlled trials. *BMJ*; **324**:1426.

Kirby, D. and Coyle, K. (1997). School-based programs to reduce sexual risk-taking behavior. *Children and Youth Services Review*; **19**:415–36.

NHS Centre for Reviews and Dissemination (1997). *Preventing and reducing the adverse effects of unintended teenage pregnancies*. NHS Centre for Reviews and Dissemination, York.

Nicoll, A., Catchpole, M., Hughes, G., Simms, I., and Thomas, D. (1999). Sexual health of teenagers in England and Wales: analysis of national data. *BMJ*; **318**:1321–2.

Public Health Laboratory Service (2002). Diagnoses of selected sexually transmitted infections (STI) in England, Wales and Northern Ireland 1991–2001.

http://www.phls.co.uk/topics_ az/hiv_and_sti/epidemiology/sti_data.htm

Scenario D
Health promotion directed at reducing motor vehicle accidents involving school-age children

Case study

Mr James, orthopaedic surgeon at St Stephen's Children's Hospital, is carrying out his ward round on a Monday morning following the weekend 'take'. On this occasion, he is accompanied by Stephen Charnley, the community paediatric trainee who has been attached to the firm. He notices that of the children on the ward who have fractures of the long bones, two live on the same street. On further enquiry, he establishes that this is one of the worst roads in the town for road traffic volume and speeding. He remembers reading in the local paper that there have been three deaths in the past year of young children crossing the road.

Background epidemiology

Childhood accidents are the top cause of death in children and are highly amenable to prevention. The chief cause of death is collision between a motor vehicle and a child pedestrian or cyclist, where the degree of trauma to the child is very great. Motor traffic continues to increase in the UK and there is insufficient protection for children.

What works?

There is considerable scope for prevention. The chief factors causing motor vehicle accidents (in which there is a large social class variation) are children playing on the streets, the lack of safe play areas—especially in areas of high social deprivation, high car speeds in residential neighbourhoods, lack of separation of cyclists, cars, and pedestrians, and the limited use of cycle helmets. Measures which can be taken to reduce risk are mainly outside the scope of the health sector. There is considerable evidence of the benefit of traffic calming, both in terms of injury reduction and in improving neighbourhood interaction (Fig. 7.1).

Other measures include promoting the use of cycle helmets, the introduction of more cycle paths, and traffic reduction policies. The latter would improve children's health in many ways, including the reduction of particulate emissions associated with respiratory infections and asthma. Evidence is building that as a result of increasing car transport by children, there is a reduction in physical fitness as a direct result of less walking or cycling opportunity.

This field is one of the most important for child health promotion, since accidents are such a high-ranking cause of death and disability and the means of preventing them are well known. Other countries have demonstrated that success is possible. There is, however, a big question of political will—hence the important role of advocacy in this area. Paediatricians and public health practitioners were successful in lobbying for child-proof containers and need to be equally forceful in relation to leglislation on traffic reduction and the separation of cyclists from cars.

Preventing unintentional injuries in children and young adolescents

+ Ensure increased availability of child car restraints (through loan schemes), smoke detectors, and cycle helmets
+ Involve target group in planning of eduational methods and use not more than one or two specific messages
+ Community programmes should be based on data derived from surveillance systems and target specific injuries and age groups
+ In the 15–24 year age range, the most effective measures are leglislative or regulatory controls
+ Advocacy for area-wide urban safety measures
+ Collaboration between agencies is important but takes time to develop

Summary of recommendations from *Effective Health Care Bulletin*, June 1996

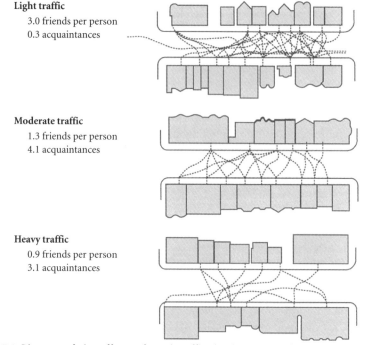

Light traffic
3.0 friends per person
0.3 acquaintances

Moderate traffic
1.3 friends per person
4.1 acquaintances

Heavy traffic
0.9 friends per person
3.1 acquaintances

Fig. 7.1 Diagram of the effects of road traffic density on social interaction (Source: Appleyard and Lintell, 1972, permission sought).

Health promotion is effective at both national and local levels. Nationally, measures might include reduction of traffic speeds in built-up areas; greater encouragement of cycle lanes; leglislation on cycle helmets, and traffic reduction legislation. At regional or district level, measures might include promotion of 'Safe Routes to School', greater creation of home zones and 20 mph limits, local school and community schemes to promote cycle helmets, local council traffic calming schemes in all residential neighbourhoods, and local congestion charging.

Who are the stakeholders?

Those with an interest include paediatricians, A&E consultants, the public health department, school nurses, the health promotion unit; transport and road safety departments in the local authority, local councillors, and parents and school governors (especially in relation to Safe Routes to School).

An approach

Stephen is aware that this can be a difficult issue to get going, despite its importance. He talks first to the local child public health lead in the Primary Care Trust (PCT) (Ms Dorothy Kenny, a former health visitor manager with a higher degree in public health) who has a special interest in this area. Dorothy is a strong supporter of Sustrans, an organization that is aiming to further develop safe routes to school, and is aware of other groups active in this area including Transport 2000 (working to reduce traffic and make roads more people friendly) and the National Children's Bureau initiative to support home zones. The local Child Accident Prevention Group has been dormant for some time, and Dorothy and Stephen decide that it would be useful to re-invigorate the group and use it as a focus for lobbying for safe routes to school, using the example of the two boys in hospital as the 'trigger'. The street the boys live on is part of a health action zone (HAZ) so that inter-agency networks have already been established locally and form the basis for the subsequent campaign.

The local school takes an active role by placing a highly visible black disc, 30 cm wide, on the nearest lamp post, for every serious accident which occurs within a half mile radius. The discs are a constant reminder to local people (and policy makers) of the dangers of traffic in the area. Using a small grant from the local authority, the school purchase high-quality cycle helmets in bulk to be sold to parents at cost. The home–school association become involved in developing a Safer Routes to School proposal and bidding for funding. The scheme is fronted by a local celebrity who has severe spinal injuries from a road traffic incident in her childhood and is wheelchair bound.

The Child Accident Prevention Group agree to meet regularly to review progress and to look at other injury prevention initiatives. It is agreed that Mr James will monitor injury rates using a monthly print-out of all fractures of the long bones and head injuries treated in the hospital. He agrees to display this in the A&E department as a map of accident 'hot spots' and to encourage hospital staff to take an active role in secondary prevention.

This is an example which originated in a hospital setting and was followed up as an active prevention outreach. Severe injuries are only the tip of the iceberg of morbidity associated with road traffic accidents but a useful place to start because of the heavy burden in terms of loss of function and time off school.

Further reading

Department of Health (2002). *Preventing accidental injury—priorities for action.* Stationery Office, London.

Duperrex, O., Roberts, I., and Bunn, F. (2002). *Safety education of pedestrians for injury prevention (Cochrane Review). The Cochrane Library, Issue 4.* Update Software, Oxford.

Marsh, P. and Kendrick, D. (1998). Injury prevention training: is it effective? *Health Education Research*; **13**:47–56.

Towner, E., Dowswell, T., Mackereth, C., and Jarvis, S. (2001). *What works in preventing unintentional injuries in children and young adolescents? An updated systematic review.* Health Development Agency, London.

Scenario E
Promotion of breast-feeding
Case study

Hilda Benson, a health visitor in a depressed Midlands town, in what was formerly a thriving coal-mining area, has a particular interest in breast-feeding. She has seen a recent government report which shows a modest increase in breast-feeding rates at birth nationally over the last few years, but with a more rapid falling-off over the first few weeks of life than in the past. She suspects from her own experience, and from talking to other health visitors in the area, that breast-feeding initiation rates locally are considerably lower than the national average of 69%. Hilda has recently been on a course which re-emphasized the value of breast-feeding and suggested ways in which health professionals can promote breast-feeding in their patch, and—fired with enthusiasm—she decides she wants to do something about this issue.

Background

Breast-feeding is known to confer substantial benefits on both mother and baby. Hilda's notes from her recent refresher course contain the following list:

Benefits of breast-feeding

Infant	Mother
Improved nutrition	Convenience and cost
Fewer gastrointestinal infections	No risk of errors in making up bottles
Fewer respiratory infections	Quicker weight loss after pregnancy
Less risk of atopic eczema, asthma, etc.	Decreased risk of breast and ovarian
Lower rates of obesity, diabetes, and	cancer
coronary heart disease in later life	
Possible decrease in risk of cot death	
Possible increase in IQ	

Hilda knows that the World Health Organisation recommends exclusive breast-feeding for the first six months, and that the UK government supports this and wants local action to promote breast-feeding. She is aware that there is a large social class divide in breast-feeding prevalence (although the most recent government report shows a greater increase in lower social classes than higher, which is encouraging). She also knows that rates vary by ethnic group, with rates as high as 95% among mothers of African and Caribbean origin, and 87% among Asian mothers, with the white population trailing behind.

Hilda is aware that the La Leche League is active in neighbouring towns. This is a voluntary organization which supports breast-feeding by befriending new mothers and offering practical advice and emotional support. There are no La Leche groups operating in her town, and little promotion of breast-feeding in the local media. The reasons for low breast-feeding rates are thought to include cultural attitudes, lack of direct contact with breast-feeding mothers, limited knowledge of the benefits of breast-feeding, and heavy media promotion of bottle-feeding. She has been told of the evidence that certain measures to support breast-feeding—such as improving mother-infant contact immediately after birth and rooming-in mother and baby together in the post-natal ward—can be beneficial, but that there is little evidence to support any specific measures to increase the prevalence of breast-feeding. Hilda has heard of UNICEF's 'Baby friendly criteria', designed to encourage hospitals to develop policies which favour breast-feeding, but she doesn't think the local maternity unit has adopted them.

UNICEF's baby friendly hospital criteria: ten steps

1. Have a written policy that is routinely communicated to all health care staff
2. Train all health care staff in skills necessary to implement the policy
3. Inform all pregnant women about the benefits and management of breast-feeding
4. Help mothers to initiate breast-feeding within half an hour of birth
5. Show mothers how to breast-feed and how to maintain lactation even if they should be separated from their infants
6. Give newborn infants no food or drink other than breast milk, unless medically indicated
7. Practise rooming-in, allowing mothers and infants to remain together 24 hours a day
8. Encourage breast-feeding on demand
9. Give no artificial teats or pacifiers to breast-feeding infants
10. Foster the establishment of breast-feeding support groups and refer mothers to them on discharge from hospital

Who are the stakeholders?

Paediatricians, hospital and community midwives, health visitors, GPs, Director of Public Health and Director of Health Improvement in the PCT, hospital trust chief executives, voluntary and community groups.

An approach

Hilda writes a short paper setting out the benefits of promoting breast-feeding locally. She points out that there is a strong likelihood of health gain if more mothers breast-feed, particularly through the reduction of enteric and respiratory infections which are known causes of mortality and morbidity in infancy. There will also be longer-term benefits for both mothers and babies, and there may be benefits to parent–child interaction, though these are not evidence-based. She includes what is known about the effectiveness of promoting breast-feeding, and sets out a few ideas for action locally.

Initially, Hilda takes the paper to the health visitors' professional forum, where there is widespread support for the idea of a local breast-feeding project. The health visitor representative on the Primary Care Trust Board agrees to take the paper to a board meeting and to pass it on to the Director of Health Improvement.

Some weeks later, Hilda hears that the PCT has agreed to make this a priority area for health promotion locally and has allocated a small amount of money for development work. The PCT is part of a Health Action Zone (HAZ), a locality receiving funds for inter sectoral development. It is decided that the work should be taken forward by a HAZ task group. Hilda agrees to chair the group, which is asked to submit a project plan. She initially recruits the following people to help her:

- a GP from the local practice who has an interest in maternal and child health
- a representative from the local branch of the National Childbirth Trust, whom she has discovered is very supportive of an initiative to increase breast-feeding
- a community midwife
- a specialist registrar in public health from the PCT.

At the first meeting of this group, it is agreed that the main difficulty in developing health promotion measures for breast-feeding is the large number of potential areas for action, and the limited evidence of effectiveness of any particular intervention. There is a clear need for more research, but little likelihood of progress in time to help this project. Evaluation of any interventions agreed by the task group will be important.

It turns out that the public health registrar has recently completed a local survey of breast-feeding, seeking information on breast-feeding prevalence at birth and six weeks, any advice which mothers were offered from different sources, and users' views about local services including the support available from midwives, health visitors, and others. The results showed that the local prevalence of breast-feeding is 60% at birth and 30% at six weeks, and that the main sources of advice cited were friends, female relatives, and the media, with midwives and health visitors rated much lower. A sizeable proportion of women felt local breast-feeding support services were inadequate and might have helped them continue breast-feeding for longer. However, another sizeable proportion said they had never considered breast-feeding.

The group agrees that they should develop proposals both for health promotion interventions to increase the initial uptake of breast-feeding, and for improving support services to help breast-feeding mothers continue for longer. They agree to consider action at national, local, and individual level, since there is always scope

Table 7.2 Breast-feeding promotion initiatives

National level
- Strategic and policy support for breast-feeding
- Positive media advertising of breast-feeding and better information for parents on its benefits
- Control of advertising of bottle-feeding
- Longer statutory maternity leave
- Guidelines for training of health professionals
- Promotion of guidelines for 'Baby Friendly' hospitals and communities
- Legislation to protect mothers' rights to breast-feed in public places
- More routine data collection on prevalence

Local level
- Local media advertising in support of breast-feeding
- Encourage adoption of 'Baby Friendly' criteria
- Staff training for all midwives, health visitors, and GPs—breast-feeding lead for each patch?
- Breast-feeding support services, including drop-in clinics, outreach, possibly helpline
- Work closely with local voluntary organizations including NCT and La Leche League
- Develop peer support network / local breast-feeding champions
- Encourage facilities for breast-feeding locally, in restaurants, shops etc.—'Baby Friendly' awards for local businesses?
- Focus on hard-to-reach groups and those with low prevalence e.g. teenage mothers, lower socio-economic groups
- Link to PHSE classes in local schools, youth clubs, etc. to educate young people about benefits of breast-feeding
- Work with fathers—believed to be a key influence
- Continuing/wider data collection on prevalence of breast-feeding

Individual level
- Advice and information on benefits of breast-feeding
- Support from professionals and peers for those initiating breast-feeding
- Support/equipment for those returning to work e.g. breast pumps

for advocacy and lobbying to affect higher-level policy. After a brainstorming session, the group produces a long list of possibilities (see Table 7.2).

Programme of action

Following their discussions, the group agrees the following preliminary programme of action:

- Appointment of co-ordinator for the project, using development money
- HAZ-wide audit of data collection and agreed standards data collection at different ages

- ◆ Encouragement of maternity hospital to apply for 'Baby Friendly' status
- ◆ Organization of training workshops for health professionals (midwives, health visitors, GPs) on how to support breast-feeding
- ◆ Local advertising (e.g. on buses) on buses of breast-feeding
- ◆ Introduction and evaluation of peer counselling schemes
- ◆ Links with NHS Direct to co-ordinate advice on breast-feeding support and management
- ◆ Work with PCTs on developing community 'Baby Friendly' initiative
- ◆ Link to 'Healthy Schools' scheme to explore possibility of including breast-feeding in the personal, social, and health education (PSHE) syllabus
- ◆ Link to teenage pregnancy task group to ensure support and advice to teenage mothers on breast-feeding
- ◆ Link to local Chamber of Commerce to explore 'Baby Friendly' businesses
- ◆ Explore scope for UNICEF community 'Baby Friendly' award for PCTs.

This proposed work programme is submitted to the PCT and HAZ for approval. Meanwhile, different members of the group agree to explore possible costs and resources for each proposal.

The task group may need to expand to include further representatives from this list, and will certainly need to keep them informed of action and progress. It is agreed that the group should produce a newsletter containing information on the benefits and prevalence of breast-feeding and updates on local action to promote it, which could be widely circulated to professionals and the public. Sponsorship for this will be sought from a local business. It is clear that there is a long way to go, but the group has made a good start in defining a framework for action.

Further reading

Cattaneo, A. and Buzzetti, R. (2001). Effects on rates of breast feeding of training for the Baby Friendly Hospital Initiative. *BMJ*; **323**:1358–62.

Dennis, C.L., Hodnett, E., Gallop, R., and Chalmers, B. (2002). The effect of peer support on breast-feeding duration among primiparous women: a randomized controlled trial. *CMAJ*; **166**:21–8.

Fairbank, L., O'Meara, S., Renfrew, M.J., Woolridge, M., Sowden, A.J., and Lister–Sharp, D. (2000). A systematic review to evaluate the effectiveness of interventions to promote breast feeding. *Health Technology Assessment*; **4(25)**.

Hamlyn, B., Brooker, S., Oleinikova, K., and Wands, S. (2002). *Infant feeding 2000*. The Stationery Office, London.

Hoddinot, P. and Pill, R. (1999). Qualitative study of decisions about infant feeding among mothers in the east end of London. *BMJ*; **318**:30–4.

Nicoll, A. and Williams, A. (2002). Breast feeding. *Archives of Disease in Childhood*; **87**:91–2.

Saadeh, R. and Akre, J. (1996). Ten steps to successful breastfeeding: a summary of the rationale and scientific evidence. *Birth*; **23**:154–60.

Sikorski, J. and Renfrew, M.J. (2000). Support for breastfeeding mothers. *Cochrane Database of Systematic Reviews*. CD001141.

Scenario F
Child health surveillance programme—delay in diagnoses
Case study

The District Child Health Surveillance Co-ordinator, Daniel Tan, has recently been involved in a medico-legal case involving a seven-year-old boy whose parents are suing the GP for late diagnosis of their son's testicular maldescent, resulting in the child having one testis much smaller than the other. This followed on closely from another medico-legal case where a child with phenylketonuria (PKU) had been diagnosed late, at the age of 18 months. These cases have occurred despite the fact that there is a district policy on early referral of undescended testes and PKU is a condition which is specifically screened for in the neonatal period. Daniel wants to look into these cases and explore the reasons for the late diagnoses.

Background

Most countries have developed preventive programmes for maternal and child health as a response to poor infant mortality or suboptimal child health status. To a greater or lesser extent these are published as national policies, albeit with regional variations. The basic elements are immunization, health education, and screening tests. Table 7.3 shows the current UK programme: the USA equivalent is the Bright Futures programme. UK policy is based on a rigorous critical review of the international literature by a multiprofessional working group.

In the UK, delivery of the programme is based in primary care, mainly in general practice and partly in community health clinics. The personnel involved often work in several different settings and are employed by different authorities.

Following the 1990 NHS reforms, preschool child health surveillance (CHS) was highlighted as an area for increased involvement of GPs. Targets were set for immunization rates, with different payment rates conditional on reaching 70% or 90% coverage. In addition, a list of practices wishing to carry out CHS was established which was held by the employing authority at the time (Family Health Services Association—FHSA). In order to be eligible for inclusion on the 'list', GPs had to establish they had sufficient competence either by holding appropriate postgraduate qualifications or by attendance at special training courses.

The professionals involved include:

◆ midwives (hospital and community)
◆ health visitors
◆ GPs
◆ community paediatricians
◆ school nurses
◆ clerical staff
◆ child health information system manager

Table 7.3 Summary of recommended UK child health surveillance programme

Age	Review and screening procedures	Immunization	Health promotion
Newborn	**Review:** Family history Pregnancy Birth **Full physical examination including:** Weight Heart & pulses Hips Birth marks Testes Head circumference plotted Eyes (exclude cataracts and squint) Guthrie test after 6 days (PKU, hypothyroidism) Sickle cell (if indicated) Cystic fibrosis **Consider:** Risk factors for hearing loss—refer to *Can your baby hear you?* in PCHR. **If high risk then refer for Oto-acoustic emission, brainstem auditory evoked response**	BCG (high risk) Hep B (if mother is a carrier)	Cot death prevention Feeding technique Nutrition Baby care Crying Sleep Car safety Family planning Passive smoking Dangers of shaking baby Sibling management

10–14 days	Guided by results and review of neonatal check Assess and establish levels of support and assistance required Review sickle cell and thalassaemia test (if appropriate)	Review BCG and Hep B status Introduce to immunization programme and obtain informed consent	Nutrition Breast feeding Passive smoking Accident prevention: bathing, scalding, and fires Explanation of tests and results Encouraging parents to request results rof all tests Significance of prolonged jaundice Depression, coping, and help (parents/carers)
6–8 weeks	**Review:** Parental concerns e.g. vision, hearing, activity Risk factors including significant family history **Full examination including:** Weight Head circumference Centile plotting Hip check Testes Eyes—red reflex, squint, movement, tone, and general development Heart and pulses Report Guthrie results back to parents	1st DT Pert Hib/Pol Meningococcal C	Immunization Nutrition and dangers of early weaning Accidents: fires, falls, over-heating, scalds Refer parent to Can your baby hear you? in PCHR Recognition of illness in babies and what to do Fever management Crying Sleeping position Passive smoking Review of car safety Depression (parents/carers)

Table 7.3 cont.

Age	Review and screening procedures	Immunization	Health promotion
2–4 months	Parental concerns	2nd & 3rd DT Pert Hib/Pol. Meningococcal C	Weighing as appropriate Maintain previous health promotion Promotion of language and social development Refer parent to *Can your baby hear you?* in PCHR Deter future use of baby walkers
6–9 months	Discussion of developmental progress, asking specifically about vision, hearing, and language development Check weight and head circumference as required or if parental concern Observe behaviour and look for squints		Parental concerns Nutrition Refer parent to *Can your baby hear you?* in PCHR Accident prevention; fires, choking, scalding, burns, stair gate, fire guard, etc. Review of transport in cars Dental care Play and development needs
13 months		1st MMR	
18–24 months	Parental concerns, behaviour, vision, and hearing Observe gait Emphasize value of comprehension and social	Review immunization status	Safety—accident prevention, falls from heights, drowning, poisoning, road safety Development—language and

	communication in relation to speech development (speech and language screening tests) Public health 'sign off'—check records to ensure full coverage of screening and immunization		play Management and behavioural issues Promote positive parenting Toilet training Diet, nutrition, prevention of iron deficiency
39–48 months	Enquiry and discussion of vision, squint, hearing, behaviour, language acquisition, development—referral as necessary Education needs and choices—notification of any special educational needs and choices Measure height and plot Check testicular descent has been recorded, if not examine Where concerns about hearing impairment, perform test (e.g. McCormick toy discrimination test) Visual acuity by orthoptist	Check immunization status DT/polio (preschool booster) 2nd MMR	Safety—accident prevention, burns, road safety, drowning, poisoning, falls from heights Development—language and play socialization Management of behaviour issues School readiness Nutrition/diet Dental care Toilet training
5 years: school entrant	Review preschool record including a check for record of testicular and heart examination School entrant review—parent and school nurse Establish teachers'/parental concerns Height (plot and compare with previous measurements), weight, and hearing sweep Visual acuity (Snellen) if not previously carried out	Review of immunization status	Obtain consent for planned programme and health checks Access to school health School health surveillance programme Sleep Friendships/settling at school Accident prevention, road safety, stranger danger

Table 7.3 *cont.*

Age	Review and screening procedures	Immunization	Health promotion
	Observation of gait and fine motor skills		Dentist, dietician Management of medicines at school Care in the sun
7–8 years (Year 3)	Teacher concerns Review of records Height, weight, vision General health check Issues raised by child		Accident prevention, road safety, safety at play, stranger danger Friendships Exercise, nutrition, and dental care Care in the sun
11–12 years (Year 7)	Visual acuity Colour vision General health check Issues raised by young person Support for individual programmes of care		Accident prevention Relationships Exercise/nutrition Smoking Dental care Management of medication in school Puberty/sexual health Care in the sun

Age			
12–13 years (Year 8)		Heaf Test BCG	
14–15 years (Year 10)	General health check including height, weight, vision (where concerns) Issues raised by young person	TB/polio booster	Substance abuse—alcohol, smoking, drugs, solvents Diet/exercise Testicular self examination, promotion of cervical cytology Sexual health Promotion of GP well woman/man check Information about health services e.g. teenage clinics, health shop Dental health Careers
15–16 years (Year 11)	Self referral—issues raised by students	Information to school leavers on need for immunizations as adult catch-up immunization	Stress management Self referral—issues raised by students.

Source: *Health for all children* (4th edition) 2002. Oxford University Press, Oxford.

Both PKU and undescended testes are relatively low prevalence conditions, as are the other key conditions for which screening is recommended: hypothyroidism, hip dysplasia, sensorineural hearing loss, and amblyopia. The performance of screening tests for these conditions have been shown, in a number of studies, to be very variable, especially for the physical and sensory impairment items. The Guthrie heel prick biochemical test (which involves taking a few drops of blood from babies on the seventh day of life, once feeding has been established, and sending it to a reference laboratory on a special piece of absorbent card to be tested for PKU and hypothyroidism) is effective, although studies have shown that the programme as a whole can be problematic unless there is good flow of information between clinicians and laboratories. Simple things such as inadequate sampling technique, postal loss or delay, or mis-identification of infants through frequent name changes can lead to a potential catastrophe for the child and family. In the USA, the identification of a new case of congenital hypothyroidism is considered a medical emergency.

Although primary care health professionals are the key target audience for delivery of this programme, there is good evidence demonstrating the effectiveness of parents in identifying a number of developmental and sensory impairments.

The District Child Health Surveillance Co-ordinator (DCHSC) is responsible for setting up a multidisciplinary group to oversee the programme as a whole and monitor its quality. The functions of such a group are listed in the box below.

Functions of the District Child Health Surveillance Co-ordinating (DCHSC) Group

1. To share ownership of the programme and to develop agreed written aims, objectives, referral guidelines, administrative processes, and training standards

2. To develop quality standards for provision of CHS in primary care and school and methods for monitoring these

3. To ensure equitable delivery of the programme and that 'hard to reach' children and those looked after are not missed by the universal programme.

4. To introduce and co-ordinate new programmes and alterations to the existing programme

5. To establish, develop, and maintain information systems

6. To facilitate consultation with parents, children, and voluntary groups in the planning and implementation of the programme

---

Who are the stakeholders?

Midwives and health visitors have a major involvement in ensuring that the screening tests are carried out but feel that they receive little information about coverage and find out about 'abnormal' findings in an unreliable and often untimely manner. Other key individuals who are involved in the child health screening activities are the child health computer clerk and administrator of the child health system, the pathology laboratory staff, and clinic nurses.

At secondary (and tertiary) care level there are paediatricians with a special interest in endocrinology and metabolic conditions and paediatric surgeons.

Parents of young children nearly all receive a personal child health record (PCHR) which highlights the various components of the child health surveillance programme along with section for professionals to record their findings. The PCHR has helped to empower parents and demystify the process of preventive care. Increasingly, children of school age are being issued with their own records to keep along with the early years' pages. This record is thus the basis of the adult patient-held health record of the future.

An approach

There is a local evidence-based policy document, adapted from the national recommendations, which specifies referral pathways for key physical problems which the programme is aimed at detecting at an early stage. There have been a number of recent training updates organized by Daniel, with good attendance and an emphasis on clinical technique and referral pathways. Daniel is aware, however, that there is a certain scepticism locally about the value of the child health surveillance programme, especially among GPs who feel they are over-examining 'normal' children.

Daniel decides to look at each incident of delayed diagnosis as a 'critical learning exercise', with a view to sharing the findings more widely. These incidents are clinical governance and risk management issues and require a similar process of 'non-blame' enquiry. He consults members of the DCHS group, which includes representatives of most professional groups involved in the surveillance programme. The notes of the children in question are collated from primary care nursing, medical and hospital records, as well as regional laboratory data. It soon becomes apparent that there has been a deviation from the expected 'pathway' in each case. In the first case, the GP had made a prompt referral for maldescent of the testis at three months, but the surgeon and clerical staff failed to arrange further follow-up. In the second, there was an error at the point of neonatal blood sampling and testing (a midwife provided insufficient blood and the retesting was delayed).

A number of actions are agreed by the DCHSC group:

- Training subcommittee to devise a staff educational session update on testicular maldescent, emphasizing the need for careful physical examination technique and prompt referral to surgical team
- Advice to parents in the PCHR to be reviewed, so that the threshold for self-referral is lowered
- Training and awareness-raising session for clerical staff who record Guthrie test results, stressing the importance of timely reporting of 'insufficient' samples (where too little blood has been collected from an individual child)
- An audit of age at orchidopexy to be carried out between the four surgeons in the hospital to help ensure concurrence with national policy recommendations and to reduce variance

Further reading

Blair, M. (2001). The need for and role of a coordinator of child surveillance/promotion. *Archives of Disease in Childhood*; **84**:1–5.

Hall, D. and Elliman, D. (2003). *Health for all children (fourth edition)*. Oxford University Press, Oxford.

Seymour, C. *et al.* (1997). Neonatal screening for inborn errors of metabolism: a systematic review. *Health Technology Assessment*; **1(11)**.

Winter, M., Balledux, M., De Mare, J., and Burgmeijer, R. (1995). *Screening in child health care—report of the Dutch Working Party on Child Health Care*. Radcliffe Medical Press, Oxford.

Scenario G
Mitigating the health impact of social deprivation
Case study

Max Sanderson, a community paediatrician in South Knowsley NHS Trust, has been asked by the Chief Executive for Oddington Park Primary Care Trust (PCT) whether he would attend a meeting to discuss the PCT's health improvement plan. The PCT has agreed that they should develop a plan to improve child health in Marton Estate, a community well known as an area of severe social deprivation. The practices in the PCT are particularly concerned about the high teenage pregnancy rates, high proportion of low birth weight babies, the high consultation rate for babies and children, and the low immunization rates.

Background

As Chapter 1 makes clear, social deprivation is an important risk factor for a range of child health problems, particularly injury, perinatal and infant mortality, preterm birth, low birth weight, congenital abnormalities, sudden infant death, child abuse, disability, and behaviour problems. Socially deprived communities suffer high levels of crime, and community members are more likely to be exposed to violence. Drugs are often a problem and teenagers are exposed to both drug taking and the opportunity to engage in illegal drug pushing. Social trust is usually low and community members are more likely to feel isolated and unsupported. Such communities often look depressing. However, deprived communities may differ from one another. Some have large populations of people from minority ethnic groups; in some, unemployment is the norm; and in some, single-parent families are very common.

There are many way of defining poverty (see Chapter 4). According to one commonly used measure—the proportion of the population living on less than half the average national income—over one in four children born in the UK are now brought up in poverty. Consistent definitions are important for measuring trends over time, but whatever measures are used it is possible to demonstrate that the proportion of children living in poverty doubled in most Western countries in the 1970s and 80s. At the beginning of the twenty-first century the UK government has begun to tackle childhood poverty and rates have begun to fall slightly.

What works?

Health promotion and disease prevention are part of Max Sanderson's job description, but in the five years since he took up his post, clinical commitments have prevented him from developing this aspect of his job—so he was pleased to be asked to the PCT's meeting, and decided that he should prepare himself by doing a little preliminary research. Searching through databases of systematic reviews in the library, he found several from well-respected sources that covered relevant interventions shown to have the potential to improve child health in deprived communities. These identified the following as being of potential benefit:

- *Injury prevention*: cycle helmet and seat belt use; smoke detectors; area-wide urban safety measures including traffic calming; pedestrian safety
- *Passive smoking*: nicotine replacement and behavioural self-help strategies for parents who smoke
- *Pregnancy and STD prevention*: sex education in schools delivered by teachers who feel at home with the subject matter and involving peer education; accessible, confidential family planning services both in GP surgeries and on an outreach basis in schools and youth centres
- *Breast feeding*: home visiting and social support
- *Social and educational consequences of social deprivation* including delinquency and school dropout: support for parents including home visiting programmes, both professional and volunteer; group parenting programmes; drop-in centres; early years education programmes; health-promoting school initiatives which take a whole-school approach.

Max was interested to read that it appeared to matter how health promotion interventions were delivered. Many seemingly valuable interventions had proved ineffective. He read that those which were developed with the community to meet needs they had identified, and where there was community involvement, were more likely to succeed. He also read that 'multifaceted' interventions (those which involved more than one approach) and multidisciplinary approaches were more effective. It appeared that the interpersonal skills and qualities of the person delivering the intervention mattered for effectiveness.

Max also decided that he should consult the local Trust's health promotion service. He thought he ought to know what was being done already. The Director told him about a range of initiatives which were happening in Marton's schools under the umbrella of the Health Promoting Schools Award Scheme. The primary school had developed bullying and behaviour management policies, and the secondary school had a very strong and well-supported drug and smoking policy. He also learned that the school nurse in the secondary school was not keen on talking to teenagers about contraception.

Max mentioned what he had learned from his trip to the library and was surprised to find that the Director was not at all impressed. She told him that that sort of evidence was not usually helpful. Did he know that the World Health Organisation had just announced that randomized controlled trials were 'inappropriate, misleading and unnecessarily expensive' in evaluating health promoting interventions? She talked about disempowerment, explaining that it was very difficult for people with no long-term prospects to care much about their future health. She explained that Marton had been on the receiving end of a whole range of well-meaning projects. Many of these had been helpful in the short term, but invariably the project worker had got another job or the money had run out, leaving the community feeling let down and highly sceptical of 'projects'. She said she felt that the areas which were most important were skills development and employment initiatives. These were empowering and helped people out of poverty. She added that it mattered a great deal who was going to undertake the work and that their skills and experience were key. She also said that whatever the PCT did they must do in conjunction with other agencies. She felt that a rapid appraisal might be a good starting point to gather information about the community's needs and concerns. She also mentioned that she had been part of a group that had put together an unsuccessful bid for a healthy living centre in Marton.

After the meeting Max reflected that although the Director had been so dismissive of the systematic review evidence, quite a lot of it seemed to concur with what she had told him.

Who are the stakeholders?

Everyone is a potential stakeholder in a community health improvement project, but many of those who could be expected to take an interest are likely to be too busy to get involved. The PCT is potentially a very important player, especially in home visiting, parental support provision, and school health service provision, and they had already expressed an interest. Local authorities need to be involved in employment and skill development initiatives as well as in early years' provision and youth centre activities. Road traffic initiatives are also the responsibility of the local authority. Social services are likely to want to get involved in initiatives which might prevent child abuse or the need for children to be 'looked after'. The police and probation service may want to help in drug and crime prevention strategies. Voluntary organizations may be the only organizations with people trained to provide certain services. Sometimes it is possible to involve local businesses in such schemes. Local authorities should know the history of any of the large number of government initiatives to improve the well-being of deprived communities, including Education Action Zones, Sure Start projects, and Health Action Zones, and the likelihood of accessing additional monies to support any initiative in Marton.

An approach

Reflecting on all that he had learned, Max decided that he should go to the meeting and express an interest in being involved. He felt that the most important thing he could bring to the meeting was an air of realism. He wanted to ensure that the PCT was planning to develop a sustainable multidisciplinary, multifaceted approach. He wondered whether people from the local authority and voluntary sector would also have been invited, and whether it would be possible to get some members of the community involved. He realized that the first step in any health improvement plan might be to identify sources of funding: perhaps the outcome might be a bid to become a 'Sure Start' area. Of one thing he was certain—if anything useful was going to come out of the PCT's health improvement plan, they were going to need to take a long-term approach.

Max reflected that he could see this initiative spanning the next ten years of his life, and that it would be novel and attractive to be part of an initiative for which he did not have to assume responsibility single-handedly. He was also aware that it was inappropriate for him to have a clear plan in mind at this stage. In this area of work, it seemed plans needed to be made jointly and his views should not be accorded priority. It might be that none of the things he thought should happen would be addressed in the first instance. However, he also felt sure that it was important for him to be there and to be seen to be supporting the initiative.

The meeting turned out to have been well set up, and most of those who Max had thought about seemed to be represented—although he drew attention to the lack of a community representative. Those present all agreed to support a health improvement project on Marton estate focussing on child health in particular. Much to Max's surprise, the financially hard-pressed PCT agreed to fund a short-term, part-time post to co-ordinate the project initially, and it was agreed that one of the local health visitors with community development training and skills should be approached to see if she would be willing to take on the post. The meeting agreed that the project would begin with a rapid appraisal. The health visitor manager agreed to manage the project and support the project worker. The group agreed to meet quarterly and to consider at their next meeting how they might go about recruiting community members onto the group.

Further reading

Acheson, D. (1998). *Independent inquiry into inequalities in health report*. The Stationery Office, London.

Arblaster, L., Lambert, M., Entwistle, V., *et al*. (1996). A systematic review of the effectiveness of health service interventions aimed at reducing inequalities in health. *Journal of Health Services Research and Policy*, 1:93–103.

British Medical Association (1999). Inequalities in child health. In *Growing up in Britain: ensuring a healthy future for our children. A study of 0–5 year olds*. British Medical Association, London.

Scenario H
Promoting vaccine uptake
Case study

Jane Farray, local GP in Durnswood, has just notified her second confirmed case of measles in a week to the local health protection team. There has not been a case since 1987 and she is concerned that this might be the beginning of a trend related to poor uptake of primary immunization resulting from recent adverse publicity about side-effects of the MMR (measles, mumps, and rubella) vaccine and its relationship to childhood autism.

A review of Jane's own practice records reveals a 76% uptake rate for MMR and a 97% uptake for other vaccines. She contacts the public health lead for communicable diseases, Sheila Tellworth, who obtains district-wide data on immunization from the local child health office, where the computerized register is held. This shows that there has been a decrease in uptake of MMR since late 1998 for the whole area and that coverage is now at critical levels for host immunity.

Background epidemiology

MMR vaccine was introduced in the UK in 1988, and led to a dramatic reduction in the incidence of these diseases (see Fig. 7.2).

Vaccination rates are very dependent on public confidence in vaccines and the perceived threat of the diseases being immunized against. There is often a fine balance, easily tipped by perceptions of adverse effects related to specific vaccines. The research reports linking pertussis (whooping cough) immunization with encephalopathy ('brain damage') resulted in a sharp decline in the uptake of immunization in the UK in the 1970s, leading to a rise in the incidence of the disease and increased infant mortality and childhood respiratory morbidity. It is estimated that it took 15 years for the effects of the 'scare' to subside and immunization rates to return to their previously high levels (see Fig. 7.3).

In that time, there were three major epidemics and many thousand children admitted to hospital with whooping cough and its complications. Dr Farray and her colleagues in Durnswood are not keen for a repeat of this trend to happen in their area.

Vaccine safety

Concerns about vaccine safety have been in existence as long as vaccines themselves. Indeed, following the Vaccine Act of 1853, there were riots in Leicester by the anti-vaccine lobby and popular cartoons of the time depicted, as a side-effect, parts of cows growing out of humans! A clear description of the true side-effects of both immunization and the disease itself is important. Table 7.4 demonstrates these side by side.

Table 7.4 Adverse events following natural measles or vaccination with MMR

Condition	Rate after natural disease	Rate after first dose of MMR
Convulsions	1 in 200	1 in 1000
Meningitis/encephalitis	1 in 2000 to 1 in 5000	Less than 1 in 1,000,000
Conditions affecting blood clotting	1 in 3000	Less than 1 in 24,000
Severe allergic response (anaphylaxis)	—	1 in 100,000
Deaths	1 in 2500 to 1 in 5000	0

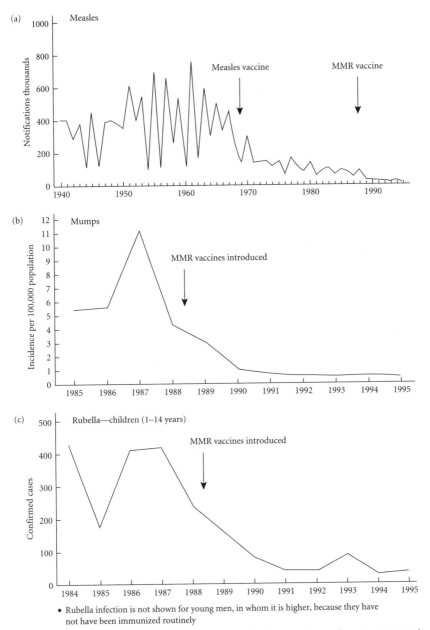

Fig. 7.2 Efficacy of vaccine introduction on the incidence of measles, mumps, and rubella.

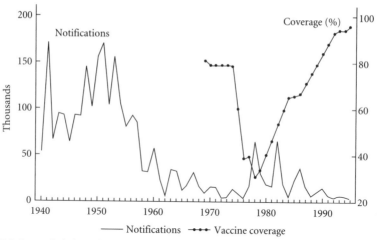

Fig. 7.3 Pertussis (whooping cough) immunization uptake and notifications of disease.

What works?

MMR vaccine is approximately 90–99% efficacious, with protection lasting between 14 and 27 years depending on the particular antigen used. Figure 7.4 demonstrates the effect of having a reduced uptake in a school population of 1000 pupils.

A review of the evidence on increasing the uptake of immunization shows the following interventions work:

• Telephone reminders to parents

• Postal reminders (linked to the child's first birthday)

• Consistent and accurate advice from health professionals

• Regular training and updating of health visitors and practice nurses on common immunization enquiries

• Written parent information which addresses common concerns

• Local immunization advisory clinic/telephone advice line

• Outreach immunization by health visitors for socially vulnerable groups (e.g. children of travelling families, those in temporary accommodation)

• Feedback of immunization uptake to practices, in a graphical form

Who are the stakeholders?

Stakeholders include parents, the district immunization co-ordinator, the anti-vaccine lobby, primary care team members, children, vaccine manufacturers, the Department of Health, local health promotion departments.

The combination of an increasingly well-educated community, the availability of multiple sources of information (and misinformation) in the media (including the

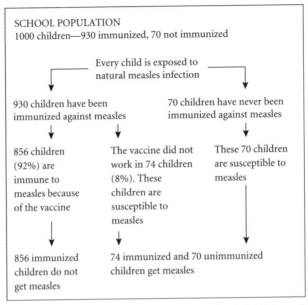

Fig. 7.4 The effects of suboptimal vaccine uptake in a school of 1000 pupils.

internet), and parents more willing to challenge medical authority, has resulted in the need for child public health professionals to become equally sophisticated in presenting the options available. A multi-dimensional approach is needed.

An approach

The district immunization co-ordinator, Dr Farray, and Dr Tellworth arrange to meet to discuss how best to tackle the problem in Durnswood. Health Promotion England (HPE) has just produced an information pack on MMR for professionals with good-quality materials for parents too. The child health system manager is able to arrange for a special reminder to be sent to the parent of each child in the district at the time of their first birthday. It is agreed that this will be sent out together with a brief and well-designed information sheet taken from data given in the HPE pack, acknowledging the main concerns of the anti-vaccine lobby and local parents.

In addition, two of the health visitors in adjoining practices decide to set up a stall at the local supermarket, with the support of the local health promotion unit, to help raise the issue of declining immunization rates and how this might affect the local population. The radio station is invited to do a piece on a local health programme, and a press release is produced by Dr Tellworth for the local free newspaper. All practice nurses and health visitors are asked to attend a compulsory training session which features the use of parent 'scripts' and role play, so that negotiation skills can be improved, in addition to acquiring clear and accurate factual information.

Outreach immunization is arranged for those children identified by the computerized child health system as being three months overdue for their MMR and where consent has been obtained already. Clear guidelines are produced for referral to the immunization clinic in the paediatric department for 'difficult' cases, but the emphasis is on empowering those responsible for vaccination to manage as much as possible in the community setting by raising the general level of expertise.

The effect of the programme is monitored on a quarterly basis, with all primary care practices receiving their immunization uptake figures in a ranked graphical display corrected for deprivation score.

Immunization is one of the most cost-effective preventive interventions available. During a period of loss in public confidence in the vaccination programme, it is especially important that concerted efforts are made by all those involved with child public health to restore the balance in favour of increased protection of the community as a whole.

Further reading

Barrett, G. and Ramsay, M. (1993). Improving uptake of immunisation. *BMJ*; **307**:681–2.

Davies, G., Elliman, D., Hart, A., Nicoll, A., and Rudd, P. (1996). *Manual of childhood infections*. W.B. Saunders.

Department of Health, Welsh Office, Scottish Office Department of Health, DHSS (Northern Ireland) (1996). *Immunization against infectious disease*. HMSO, London.

Peckham, C., Bedford, H., Seturia, Y., and Ades, A. (1989). *The Peckham Report National Immunisation Study: factors influencing immunisation uptake in childhood*. Action for the Crippled Child, London.

Scenario I

Reviewing the system for investigating suspected child deaths from abuse

Case study

Anya Clegg is the newly appointed designated nurse for child protection for Sidborough North Primary Care Trust (PCT), which covers a population of 200,000 in the city centre and northern suburbs of a large town in East Anglia. She is concerned to discover that there have been two deaths of children on the child protection register within the PCT area in the last 18 months. During her first few weeks in post, she obtains copies of the serious case review ('Part 8' review) reports for each of these children in order to find out more about these specific cases and about the workings of the local child protection system and the Area Child Protection Committee (ACPC).

Details of cases

Case 1 was a baby aged six months whose mother was a known drug misuser. The baby had been subject to a pre-birth child protection case conference, and he and his two older siblings (aged two and four) were on the child protection register for actual neglect. One previous sibling had died on the special care baby unit after being born prematurely and being small for its date; a much older sibling, born when the mother was 15, had been long-term fostered and eventually adopted and was not in contact with the family. The mother had an abusive partner and the children had spent a good deal of time with their maternal grandparents, but this relationship had diminished since the new baby was born. The mother was in contact with a drug worker and had been on methadone, but admitted to having increased her heroin use again recently.

The baby died while co-sleeping with his mother on a sofa. At post-mortem he was found to be significantly underweight and to have a few superficial bruises which the mother attributed to rough treatment from his siblings, but there were no other findings suggestive of abuse and the cause of death was found to be sudden infant death syndrome (SIDS). The pathologist was aware that the child had been on the child protection register but had been given no further details of the family circumstances. The social worker in charge of the case had visited two days before the baby's death and found the mother cheerful and the baby clean and apparently well-cared for, but he reported that the flat was 'in a tip as usual', that the older children were inadequately clothed, and that the mother's partner had behaved threateningly when he questioned the mother about the children's welfare. The health visitor had also seen the mother and baby recently when she brought him for his final primary immunizations; she had been quite concerned about his weight and a skin rash and had suggested the mother took him to the GP, but had not yet got in touch with the social worker because she was new in post and unclear about how to contact him. The police had attended the scene of death, but because of a mix-up over communication no sample had been obtained from the mother for a drug screen immediately after the baby's death.

The Part 8 review concluded that professional practice in this case had been appropriate and in line with agreed protocols, and that no acts or omissions by staff could have contributed to the baby's death. It made recommendations about record keeping, communication, staff training and supervision, and other issues, which had been followed up at six-monthly intervals by the ACPC. The Coroner was satisfied with the post-mortem report and pronounced that death had been due to natural causes, without holding an inquest.

Anya was concerned that the possible role of neglect in this baby's death had not been adequately considered. She knew that co-sleeping with a parent on a sofa increased the risk of SIDS, especially if the parent smoked or had recently drunk alcohol or taken drugs. She felt the baby's physical condition was indicative of neglect, and that this too had increased his risk of SIDS. Overall, she was concerned about the level of communication between staff in different agencies, both before and after the baby's death.

Case 2 was a seven-year-old with epilepsy and learning difficulties. He had been entered on the child protection register as at risk of physical harm six months before, following an incident in which his father had pushed his mother down the stairs and the child also suffered extensive bruising. His father was, however, currently in prison on remand following a brawl in a pub in which a teenage boy had been stabbed. His mother had been diagnosed as depressed since this event and had been finding it increasingly difficult to manage her son alone. The week before, she had taken the child to the Emergency Department after he had apparently fallen off a chair, but his injuries were insignificant on that occasion and consistent with the story. The social worker had been informed and had visited soon after; her main concern was the mother's mental health, and she had been trying to arrange respite care for two nights a week. A review case conference was due to take place in four weeks' time and the social worker discussed with her supervisor the possibility of altering the category of registration, since physical harm no longer seemed the greatest risk to the child. She had written to the community paediatrician caring for the child and asked whether he would review the boy before the case conference. The special school he attended had noticed no change in his condition or behaviour: his epilepsy had been well controlled for the last year and he had had no fits in school for some time.

The child had apparently been found dead in his bed by his mother when she went to get him up one morning. She said he had shown no signs of ill health the evening before and she had not heard him wake in the night. She admitted, however, taking a double dose of the sleeping tablets recently prescribed by her GP. The physical and post-mortem findings indicated that the cause of death was acute asphyxia. The pathologist discussed the case with the community paediatrician. They agreed that the findings were consistent with accidental asphyxia during a seizure, and that this fitted in with the child's history, although it was impossible to distinguish this cause of death from asphyxia due to other causes, including deliberate smothering.

Again, the Part 8 review had found that no aspect of professional practice in this case had a bearing on the child's death, although it again made extensive recommendations, many of them along very similar lines to those from Case 1. An inquest was held in this case and an open verdict was recorded, but the Coroner was at pains to point out that this implied no criticism of the mother but simply reflected the fact that the post-mortem findings were not clear enough to be sure whether this death was accidental or from natural causes.

Anya was concerned about this case too. She knew that children with disabilities were at greater risk of abuse, and she felt the mother's mental health problems and the 'cry for help' the week before the child's death, when he was taken to casualty with a minor injury, had not been taken sufficiently seriously. Although the Part 8 review's recommendations did address these issues, Anya felt that the question of whether or not the mother had deliberately smothered the child—or indeed had not heard him fitting in the night because she had taken an excessive dose of sleeping pills—had not been faced squarely. She was also not clear that the recommendations from the Part 8 review had made any real difference to professional practice locally: the monitoring reports seemed to her to be a bureaucratic exercise.

Anya subsequently examined six further Part 8 reviews conducted within the ACPC's area in the last five years. Many of them raised the same issues and concerns—and the recommendations were depressingly familiar in each. Anya talked to a few colleagues in health and social services who admitted that they were worried about how well child deaths were managed and reviewed locally, about whether lessons were appropriately learned from them, and about broader issues of inter-agency working. Several pointed to the existence of detailed and cumbersome protocols, and to concerns about confidentiality, to explain the reluctance of staff to share sensitive information. Some also said there had been other deaths and near misses locally which they felt should have been reviewed, but that they had no channel for proposing this.

Who are the stakeholders?

A wide variety of health professionals in both hospital and community settings, including health visitors, GPs, paediatricians, A&E staff, the local public health department, social workers and the social services department, teachers and the local education department, the police family protection unit, the probation service, the Coroner, the NSPCC, and paediatric pathologists. Many of these will be represented on the Area Child Protection Committee.

An approach

At the next ACPC meeting, there was an item on the agenda about a recent report from the NSPCC concerning child deaths from abuse and neglect. The NSPCC representative introduced this, pointing out that the NSPCC believes at least half of such deaths are never identified, and that lessons are not adequately learned from them. He reminded the committee about a high-profile case which had been in the news recently and suggested that there may be greater scrutiny of local practice in future. Anya took this opportunity tentatively to share her findings from looking at local Part 8 reviews, and there were many nods round the table and a general agreement that this was not an area which was well managed locally. Anya offered to convene a subgroup to look at the issues in more detail, and this suggestion was gratefully accepted.

Anya's group included representatives from each of the ACPC member agencies: the community paediatrician, who is also designated doctor for child protection; the public health consultant responsible for child protection in the PCT; a senior education social worker; the social services lead for child protection; the Detective Inspector from the Police Family Protection Unit; a senior probation officer; and the NSPCC representative. They developed a project plan which was subsequently approved by the ACPC and involved a literature search for information on universal child death review teams (which the NSPCC representative says are well-established in the USA) and an evaluation of the local child death review system. This will comprise interviews with a range of local stakeholders (including those on the subgroup, the local coroner, the paediatric pathologist, and the hospital social workers) and an examination of local child deaths' data. Anya agreed to undertake this work jointly with the public health consultant. The main sources of local data are the public health mortality file (which contains details of all deaths) and the coroner's records (which he agrees to allow Anya access to). She also makes contact with the Foundation for the Study of Sudden Infant Deaths.

Findings

Two months later, a special ACPC meeting is convened to consider the findings from this project and agree recommendations for action. The main findings are:

- Around half of child deaths locally are referred to the coroner, and about two-thirds of these have an inquest. However, the findings are not routinely shared with other agencies.

- Only a tiny fraction of deaths have any multi-agency review, although in addition to the Part 8 review process, a Sudden Unexpected Death in Infancy Review Group has recently been established which looks at unexpected deaths under a year of age.

- Part 8 reviews locally are only conducted on children dying while on the child protection register or looked after by the local authority; 'near misses' are not included. The Department of Health guidance in *Working together to safeguard children* suggests a wider range of cases should be considered.

- Stakeholders expressed concern and confusion about a range of issues, including communication and joint working, the conduct of Part 8 reviews, suspicious deaths which are not reviewed, the impact of reviews on local practice, and the ACPC's advocacy and leadership role.

- The literature review yielded a wealth of information on child death review systems, most of it from the USA and Australia—but few such systems have been formally evaluated, so there is little evidence about their effectiveness. However, there is a consensus of expert opinion in favour of a more universal and systematic approach in which every child death is considered by a multi-agency team.

- Although child death review teams have not been formally established in the UK, a couple of examples of pilot inter-agency child death protocols are found which offer a possible way forward, providing a framework for the investigation and review of all unexpected deaths.

Next steps

A number of recommendations are agreed with the ACPC. These cover the following areas:

1. A thorough review of local practice in relation to the arrangements for and impact of Part 8 reviews.

2. The need to define explicit objectives and quality standards for the management and review of child deaths locally.

3. Consideration by member agencies of the feasibility of introducing a child deaths protocol similar to the examples Anya has found.

4. An emphasis on improving inter-agency communication, including training for all staff on confidentiality and the Children Act, and specific policies for communication in particular circumstances (e.g. ensuring the pathologist has adequate information before conducting a post-mortem, that all staff have a route for raising concerns about suspicious deaths with the ACPC, and developing better links with the coroner).

5. Agreement that culture change is needed as well as practical change—that the ACPC needs to develop a more proactive leadership and communication role; that all agencies need to re-establish a focus on child-centred, collaborative working; and that a balance needs to be struck between the safeguards offered by protocols and procedures, and the need to allow staff freedom to exercise their professional judgements in difficult situations.

There is a great deal of energy, enthusiasm, and commitment at this meeting, and Anya feels pleased to have made progress in clarifying the problems and engaging other stakeholders, and in having agreed actions with the ACPC as a whole. She is aware, however, of the danger that other issues will emerge and divert attention from this work, and that she and others will have to work hard to maintain the momentum established at the outset.

Further reading

Department of Health, Home Office, and Department for Education and Employment (1999). *Working together to safeguard children*. The Stationery Office, London.

Fleming, P. *et al*. (2000). *Sudden unexpected deaths in infancy: the CESDI SUDI Studies 1993–6*. The Stationery Office, London.

NSPCC (2001). *Out of sight: NSPCC report on child deaths from abuse 1973–2000* (2nd edition). NSPCC, London.

Reder, P. and Duncan, S. (1999). *Lost innocents: a follow-up study of fatal child abuse*. Routledge, London.

Sinclair, R. and Bullock, R. (2002). *Learning from past experience—a review of serious case reviews*. Department of Health, London.

Scenario J
Obesity: a public health strategy
Case study

Julie Birchcroft is the Minister of Public Health in the reforming government of the UK which is attempting to co-ordinate health policy across all sectors. There are political pressures to improve the health of teenagers in view of the worrying statistics on teenage pregnancy, conduct disorder, and youth crime, and Julie has been reviewing data on the health of this age group. She has been warned of the long-term problems associated with obesity in relation to adult health, especially the economic effects in terms of loss of employment. She is also aware that relationships with the food industry make this a political "hot potato", and that there has been little or no progress with anti-obesity measures in the USA. Julie feels that the first step should be an expert working party to establish evidence-based approaches to public health policy on obesity reduction.

Background epidemiology

Obesity is increasing in prevalence globally in both adults and children. This increase has been most notable in the USA where a visitor quickly notices the size of people of all social classes and relates this to the large portions of food served in restaurants and the frequency of snacking, as well as to the difficulties of getting round by any means but by car. Europe is catching up on the USA, with the UK leading in terms of the increasing fatness of its population—the increase in the UK parallels that of the USA (see Chapter 1). Eastern European countries and Germany are also seriously affected, while Northern Europe is doing much better. The obesity epidemic is also severe in Australasia.

In the UK it has been shown that obesity starts early. Among three- to four-year-old English children, during the period between 1989 and 1998, there was a 60% increase in the prevalence of being overweight (those having a body mass index > 85th centile) and a 70% increase in the prevalence of obesity (body mass index > 95th centile). This gives a clear message about when prevention should be initiated. However, not all overweight children will become overweight adults.

The effects of obesity in adult life are well known and are shown in the box below.

Health effects of obesity in adults

- Type 2 diabetes
- Cardiovascular disease and stroke
- Hypertension
- Cancers, particularly of the intestine and reproductive system
- Osteoarthritis and other joint disease
- Back pain
- Skin conditions
- Time off work
- Psychological effects

In children, the main effects are psychosocial, including social isolation, bullying, and low self-esteem, with resultant lower levels of academic attainment. Type 2 diabetes is now being seen in children also.

Whilst it is clear that there is an increase in obesity and that this is linked to changes in society, the causes of the increase are debated. Likely causes are the ready availability of energy-dense foods and the development of a snacking culture, and reduced physical activity as a result of time spent watching TV, the dominance of the car, and a reduction in school sports facilities and time for games in the curriculum. Fear of strangers has led to parents being unwilling to allow their children to travel independently. Although there is not a consensus on the relative importance of these various influences, in children the evidence points to the lack of physical activity as a key factor. It is clear that although the causes of obesity are heterogeneous—genetic predisposition, illness, and sexual abuse—the final pathway is eating too much or doing too little.

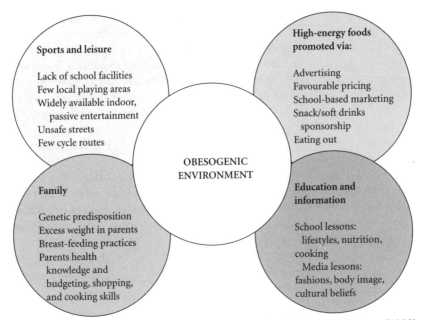

Fig. 7.5 An obesogenic environment. (Source: International Obesity Task Force (2002). With permission from Neville Rigby OTF.)

The International Obesity Task Force (IOTF) describes an obesogenic environment in Fig. 7.5.

What works?

There is very limited evidence in relation to the prevention of obesity in young people at a population level. Breast-feeding is thought to reduce the risk of obesity. It is known that individual approaches to obesity reduction are difficult to implement without very good motivation on the part of the child, which is often not present. For this reason a population-based approach is favoured, but because of the nature of our profit-oriented society, it is extremely difficult to put many of the possible policies into practice. The tendency is to say there is not enough evidence, but the "precautionary principle" would suggest that measures should be taken to target the obesogenic factors listed above.

As the IOTF 'Obesity in Europe' paper states, Ministries of Health need to:

> move away from the current ineffective approaches based on opting for 'health education'. Instead, a more structured approach to identifying the various forces and processes underlying the current 'toxic environment' is needed. This will require cross-sector collaboration with other Ministries.

There will be resistance to implementing measures directed at lifestyle factors. Whilst many people accept the potential harm of junk foods and are critical of the heavy advertising of such foods in the media, there are also very many people (particularly young people) who enjoy these foods and resist restrictions imposed both on individual choice and on corporate activity. Foods are a much harder target than tobacco for legislation because of the unending arguments about what is and what is not healthy. As with global warming, companies who profit from food consumption have clouded the picture in order to avoid any restriction of their activities. For example, any suggestion that sugar might damage health leads to heavy lobbying by the sugar industry to prove the opposite. The length of time it has taken to restrict tobacco advertising, despite very good evidence against it, suggests that it could take even longer to do the same thing with food.

Declining levels of exercise in children are related to the growth of motor traffic (the convenience of which has made it very important to a large section of the population) and to television watching (which is a popular pastime and one which many parents see as desirable). As parents themselves become less active, they are less inclined to participate in exercise with their children.

Policies which are generally accepted to have the greatest chance of success in preventing obesity at population level are listed below.

At local level (e.g. community/school)

- Whole-school approaches to improve nutrition, and nutritional standards for school meals
- Support of farmers' markets and other means to increase availability and reduce costs of healthy foods, especially fruit and vegetables
- Increase in physical activity in the school curriculum
- Provision of better sports facilities in schools and in the community
- Development of Safer Routes to School programmes, which encourage walking or cycling to school
- Development of local cycle routes and facilities, and promotion of walking and cycling
- Education on reducing time spent watching television
- Improving street safety for families

At national level

- Legislation aimed at the food and agricultural industry on fat content of meat and dairy products
- Food pricing policies
- Better labelling of nutritional content of food
- School fruit scheme
- More funding of sports facilities and support for sport and physical activity in schools
- Legislation to restrict marketing of unhealthy foods aimed at children, both in the media and in schools

- Road traffic reduction measures
- Funding for public transport and cycling, and environmental policies to support walking and cycling
- Support for Safer Routes to School programmes
- Promotion of breast-feeding

Who are the stakeholders?

There are many groups in society with the potential to influence the development of obesity, including farmers, the food industry, child health professionals, educationalists, the physical activity industry (e.g. leisure companies), and the transport sector. There are real political issues arising from the influence on government of food marketing corporations who invest large sums of money in persuading parents and children to purchase their products. The position of the government in maintaining a 'level playing field' will be crucial, but it is suspected that the reformist party which is in power is inclined to favour the interests of corporations over the public. The press also has a part to play and may attack government approaches which seem to restrict adults' ability to make their own choices on what they eat.

An approach

What, then, is the most effective approach to tackle the national epidemic of obesity? In the absence of good evidence, and with a political climate of opposition to the 'nanny state', it is unlikely that a strong public health policy response will be forthcoming, though other European countries have been more successful in this respect.

Julie decides to establish a working party which includes members of the medical Royal Colleges, voluntary organizations, Department of Health, the Food Standards Agency, ministries concerned with farming and food, and representatives from the food industry. The group's initial recommendations include the following:

- Better provision of information on the calorie content of all foods through labelling and related measures
- More emphasis on nutrition in schools through the National Curriculum
- A 'Nutrition Czar' appointed by the government to promote public education on healthy eating
- Sport England to be given additional funding for coaching facilities—but no new funding for school recreation
- Further support for the Safer Routes to School initiative, to extend this to more schools
- No action on media advertising and food pricing until further evidence is available
- Agricultural industry to investigate means of producing lower fat products
- A national monitoring exercise to track the development of obesity and establish the critical ages for its development
- A restriction on vending machines in school premises

The report is inevitably a compromise. It is also met with considerable opposition from the tabloid press, who oppose changes in farming practice which will involve further subsidies and resent further advice to the public on food issues on the grounds that 'people know what's good for them'. Headteachers create an outcry about the restriction on food vending machines, since they make a considerable profit which accrues to school funds. The voluntary sector criticizes the report for having no teeth and for failing to curb the marketing policies of the food industry. In particular, they recommend legislation to curtail the marketing of all convenience foods on children's TV—an approach which was not supported by the working party because it was not evidence-based.

Julie is moved from her post as Minister of Public Health to become Culture Minister the month after the report is issued. As a result, little action is taken and the following year the monitoring exercise (the only aspect to be implemented) demonstrates a further rise in obesity in 12–14 year-old children.

Footnote

Readers are encouraged to develop this scenario and to propose their own approach to the public health prevention of obesity, which could make a genuine difference, but is also feasible in the real world. Such an approach is likely to require considerable political lobbying by a group independent of the food industry.

Further reading

Bundred, P., Kitchiner, D., and Buchan, I. (2001). Prevalence of overweight and obese children between 1989 and 1998: population-based series of cross-sectional studies. *BMJ*; **322**:326.

Campbell, K., Waters, E., O'Meara, S., Kelly, S., and Summerbell, C. (2002). *Interventions for preventing obesity in children (Cochrane review). The Cochrane Library, Issue 4*. Update Software, Oxford.

Dietz, W.H. (2001). The obesity epidemic in young children. *BMJ*; **322**:313–14.

Dietz, W.H. and Gortmaker, S.L. (2001). Preventing obesity in children and adolescents. *Annual Review of Public Health*; **22**:337–53.

Ebbeling, C.B., Pawlak, D.B., and Ludwig, D.S. (2002). Childhood obesity: public health crisis, common sense cure. *Lancet*; **360**:473–82.

Edmunds, L., Waters, E., and Elliott, E. (2001). Evidence-based management of childhood obesity. *BMJ*; **323**:913–19.

International Obesity Task Force and European Association for the Study of Obesity (2002). *Obesity in Europe: the case for action*. EASO, London.

NHS Centre for Reviews and Dissemination (1997). The prevention and treatment of obesity. *Effective Health Care Bulletin*; **3**(2).

Reilly, J.J., Dorosty, A.R., and Emmett, P.M. (1999). Prevalence of overweight and obesity in British children: cohort study. *BMJ*; **319**:1039.

Robinson, T.N. (1999). Reducing children's television viewing to prevent obesity: a randomised trial. *JAMA*; **282**:1561–7.

World Health Organisation (1997). *Preventing and managing the global epidemic*. WHO, Geneva.

Conclusion

This chapter illustrates how problems may present in many different ways—a concern voiced by members of the local community or a professional, via the media describing a critical incident, or as a result of national policy or local funding opportunities.

Case studies in clinical practice are designed to help inform the practitioner on how best to manage another patient with a similar problem or to illustrate a particular principle which is more generalizable. We hope the examples in this chapter provide some ideas on how to manage a particular child public health issue and perhaps a few general principles which may be useful in dealing with other areas. The framework we have used for structuring the 'problems'—assessing the epidemiology of the issue and evidence base for intervention, identifying the stakeholders, and agreeing an action plan—is the starting point. The subsequent management and monitoring of progress which goes with it is akin to regular review in clinic and is just as important. Both processes have in common that professionals may facilitate and initially manage the process, but the patient or the wider community are ultimately responsible for making it happen and sustaining the desired outcomes.

Index